INTERMITTENT FASTING 101

COMPLETE GUIDE FOR BEGINNERS. A NEWBIES COURSE FOR WOMEN, MEN, AND PEOPLE OVER 50, WITH ALL YOU NEED TO KNOW TO PROMOTE HEALTH AND WEIGHT LOSS THROUGH AUTOPHAGY.

By

ROSANNE MILLER

Table Of Contents

Introduction

Just what is intermittent fasting? Although it's described as a diet, intermittent fasting is not a diet but an eating pattern that involves alternating between periods of abstaining from food and caloric drinks and fasting within a specified period. Simply put, when you follow intermittent fasting, you will be required to only eat during specific times. Intermittent fasting offers a new approach to planning your meals while tapping into the health benefits that come along with it. There are three states of intermittent fasting; the feeding state that begins right when you start eating lasting up to three to five hours during digestion and absorption. This is followed by the post-absorptive state that lasts up to 12 hours where the body doesn't process any food. Lastly, the body enters the fasting state that begins at least nine to twelve hours after your last meal. This is the time when all manner of changes and processes take place.

Naturally, most people tend to gravitate around having at least three large meals and at most six small meals. Intermittent fasting offers a departure from this because you're consciously opting to stay without food for a specified duration. Thus, you can either miss breakfast daily making lunch your first meal of the day. I'm sure you have been made to believe that breakfast is the most important meal of the day and you should in no way skip it. Well, this pattern of eating goes against such myths without putting you in harm's way.

When doing intermittent fasting, you'll need to establish your fasting and feasting windows and stick to them. This decision should be made taking into account your lifestyle and the ease of implementing it. For instance, if you're in a labor intensive job, you'll do well to align your feasting window to your work hours so that you are well energized for the day. You need to keep in mind that unlike many diets that dictate the kind of foods you need to eat, intermittent fasting doesn't have such restrictions. Instead, you can eat the foods you'd normally eat only that you must be careful not to indulge in the junk.

History of Intermittent Fasting

When you hear about intermittent fasting, you may think that it's a completely new phenomenon but you're wrong. Fasting has been practiced by many generations long before the industrial revolution. However, this was not voluntary because it was necessitated by a lack of adequate food. Ancient civilizations that mainly comprised of hunters and gatherers who didn't have a sophisticated way of preserving food. Therefore, they ate as much as they could during times of plenty and fasted when food was scarce. Although not intentional, they fasted for days depending on the time of the year and when they would find food.

Ancient Greeks too caught up with the benefits of intermittent fasting and embraced it long before scientific research was done. The Greeks believed that fasting has the ability to improve concentration and cognitive abilities. On the other hand, one of America's founding fathers Benjamin Franklin wrote, "The best of all medicines is resting and fasting." Fasting has also been practiced in different religions around the world with the concept being the same; you set aside a period during which you will not eat anything. The Father of Medicine, Augustin Hippo also recognized the value of fasting by stating "To eat when you're sick it to feed your illness". He held the belief that by fasting you're allowing the body to heal itself.

British journalist Michael Mosley popularized intermittent fasting when he shared the benefits he obtained from the 5:2 intermittent fasting protocol. It's then that this diet began to gain traction and continues to be popular to date. Today, there are different ways of doing intermittent fasting that is suitable for your convenience and preference.

How Does Intermittent Fasting Work?

When you skip meals over a specified period, your caloric intake reduces significantly and after a while, your body enters a fasted state after a while. This means that your body has used up all the fuel that was available and has now turned to the stored fuel in the form of body fat for energy. During fasting, hormones are released signaling the body to take advantage of the fat stores as opposed to tapping energy from glycogen by eating food. Intermittent fasting helps to trigger this process thus contributing to weight and fat loss alongside many other health benefits you'll experience

The Science Behind Intermittent Fasting

Your body responds differently when you eat and when you fast. When you eat, digestion takes place within a couple of hours with the fuel produced being used as energy while the surplus is stored as energy in the form of fat. On the contrary, when you fast, the body taps into the stored energy (fat) for fuel resulting in significant weight loss. Fasting also triggers the production of growth hormones thus giving your muscles a major boost. Fasting often triggers a growth hormone response that is critical in the prevention of loss of muscle.

Chapter 1.
An introduction to intermittent fasting

What is Intermittent Fasting

Intermittent fasting (IF) When most people hear this concept they disregard it and assume it sounds to complex or that they wouldn't be able to manage it. Some of the common things I often hear are:

"What the hell… not eating? I will go into starvation mode!"

"But I have to keep my metabolic fire stoked and burning to lose fat!"

"You're stupid Peter… there is no way that's healthy."

However these people forget that every single day of their lives they have been practicing intermittent fasting on some level. What do I mean by this? Well, when you sleep you fast and when you're awake you eat – this is intermittent fasting. These people are often usually undereducated on the topic and haven't studied just how beneficial it is.

The fitness industries approach to IF just takes this further by increasing the window of fasting and decreasing the window of eating. At its core level the practice of intermittent fasting is very simple - do not let this fool you though as once you explore the area deeper it becomes highly complex. In this book I will take the complex data, scientific results and theories and break it all down into a simple, easy to understand format.

In the past few years IF has become increasing popular gaining raving endorsements from bodybuilders, models, athletes and celebrities such as Hugh Jackman and Beyoncé. This explosion in popularity of IF is in no way surprising as once you start your IF journey you will see an incredible array of results.

The increasing popularity of IF is, in my mind, due to two main factors:

- The extensive list of powerful benefits it delivers

And

- The ease of which it can be adopted and maintained.

This is crucial as it has been shown that most diets and dieters fail because of two main barriers. These barriers are the complexity of managing a diet and the time they take to show results. How often have you heard someone wondering if "eating this food will negatively affect my diet" or "I've been on diet XYZ for 2 weeks now and I'm not seeing the results I want!"

Intermittent fasting knocks clean through these barriers with its simple, easy to follow procedures and its speed of results.

The concept of IF goes against much of what the fitness and health industry has long believed but as this book will detail – just because something is popular and repeated by everyone and their grandma's it doesn't mean it's true.

Common Fitness and Nutrition Myths

In the early days of its arising intermittent fasting came under a huge amount of scrutiny as it goes against everything that has been taught in the fitness industry for the past 50 years.

The concept of purposefully not eating is, at first appearances, a fitness fallacy. However once you explore the idea and challenge the past assumptions with scientific data you begin to see some shocking things.

I first off want to explore and debunk possibly the most well-known and quoted dietary "fact". This "fact" stands in the way of many people accepting the benefits of IF and is often quoted when criticising IF.

1. "You have to eat 5-6 small meals a day to keep your metabolism burning."

Unless you have lived under a rock for the past two decades I'm sure you've heard this from absolutely everyone. It is one of those rare pieces of advice that spreads like wildfire and is adopted by every-single-person. This advice has become so popular it has basically been adopted as a rock-solid fact.

However it is a lie, with zero scientific evidence to support it. That's right, one of the most well-known pieces of fitness and health advice is false.

The logic behind this theory is that eating small meals continually throughout the day will cause you to burn more fat. This comes from the idea that as eating increases your metabolic rate, eating frequently will keep your metabolic rate increased. Unfortunately this has never been proven, despite the fact that many studies have tried – and failed.

As is always the case with scientific research whilst some groups are trying to prove a theory, others are trying to disprove it. For this theory of frequent feeding, the teams disproving it won and multiple papers have been published on the topic. The most famous of which is a paper entitled:

"Increased Meal Frequency Does Not Promote Greater Weight Loss."

A team of Canadian researchers disproved the model of frequent feeding and detailed that it doesn't actually matter when or how often you eat, rather it is the amount you eat.

I want to note here that you can lose weight eating 6 small meals but it is not the frequency of eating or the meal timing that is the weight loss driver. Instead it is the amount you eat – small meals usually result in lower caloric intake.

Now for another piece of nutritional and fitness advice that has been touted by everyone for many years…

2. "Breakfast is the Most Important Meal of the Day"

This seemingly makes perfect sense and does have some inherent benefits to it, however it is not necessarily true and there is scores of evidence to disprove it. I am not saying breakfast is bad, wrong or that you should avoid it… I am simply noting that just because it is popular doesn't make it right and that there are more effective strategies.

The concept of breakfast being the most important meal of the day is that it helps you start the day, gives you energy and fuels your day. Now while these points have value to them, you have to remember most people make poor dietary choices at breakfast. These choices actually result in the opposite of the touted benefits occurring.

Combined with this is the idea that eating food (particularly carbohydrates) later in the evening will cause you to gain fat - this is another common myth that science has disproven. In actuality later feeding can result in some of the following benefits: increase in fat loss, increase in testosterone, better sleep and an increase in muscle gain.

There are benefits to not eating later in the evening but the evidence points to the benefits of eating later as outweighing the benefits of eating earlier.

Practices of IF usually suggest skipping breakfast, I will explore this in more detail later.

3. "Eat THIS, not that!"

Another fitness and nutritional staple is that you must eat certain foods and follow a specific diet in order to achieve your goals.

Whether your goals are weight loss, gaining muscle or living a longer and healthier life every guru, nutritionist and personal trainer will espouse his or her preferred diet as the ONLY way to achieve your goals.

Some of the common diets you may have been told to follow are:

- Low carb, high protein, zero fat

- High Fat, high protein zero carb

- Slow-carb diet

- DASH diet

- Palaeolithic

- Carb cycling

- Atkins

There are literally hundreds of different diets you could follow, each of them have pros and cons but what I often find is that they all fall short in one area – how easy it is to stick to them.

Sure each of these diets will help you achieve your goals but no matter how effective a diet is, if you don't stick to it religiously you will negatively impact your progress. When you lock yourself into a specific diet you limit your choices and make it very hard to follow it – this results in failed dieting.

Intermittent fasting will circumvent this as it doesn't promote any particular diet style, instead it suggests a change in your eating frequency and window. Yes, there are some guidelines to follow but these are very loose and for the most part you can eat whatever type of foods you like.

Chapter 2.
The basics of intermittent fasting

When you're eating a balanced meal, you want to eat a lot of fruits and vegetables. This is your fiber. Then add some protein, healthy fats, and grains. Combining fiber and protein with every meal means that you'll feel full longer. It will satiate your hunger hormone and help you during your fasting window. Let's look at an example of what your meals could be. Half of your plate should be vegetables of fruit. About one-third of your plate should be grains, preferably whole grains or starchy vegetables. Protein like tofu, fish, meat, and beans should fill the rest of your plate, a little less than one-fourth of your plate. This is how a balanced meal looks. To add dairy, have some on the side or as a snack. It can also be a great breakfast choice. For dairy, choose fat-free or low-fat options.

Try to avoid processed foods because they have a lot of sugar and carbs that are more than you need. It's also hard to measure them as part of a well-balanced meal. A well-balanced meal doesn't mean that you need to count calories. Instead, what you're looking at is food that will keep you full but also give you good nutrients.

Well-Balanced Breakfast Ideas

Whether your breakfast will be small or large, once you break your fast, you want to try to mix protein and fiber. Record what you eat and write down how your body feels after eating it. This will help you know what works for breaking your fast and what doesn't work. Some people react negatively to eating sugars and carbs in the morning, so keep track of your reactions to these items. Here are some breakfast ideas that give you a good mix of fiber and protein.

1. Hot oatmeal with fruit, nuts, and yogurt: This is a great mix of fiber from oatmeal and fruit, healthy fats from nuts, and dairy/protein.

2. Whole-grain toast and peanut butter/almond butter: Have a side of fruit to eat with it. Try one cup of blueberries or an apple. Or if you want to get crazy, slice some bananas and put them on your peanut butter toast.

3. Whole-grain cereal with one cup of milk: Milk gives you your protein, and whole-grain cereal is your fiber. Some people may not find this filling enough after ending a fast. If you're still hungry, add some fruit or nuts to eat with the cereal. Make sure you read the list of ingredients on the cereal box. Some cereals claim to be "whole grain," but they're often not. Choose one that will give you good fiber content.

4. Eggs and whole-grain toast: Add a side of vegetables if you want to make a larger breakfast. Think avocados for their healthy fat or try tomatoes and peppers.

5. Yogurt and granola: Granola are a carb and is sugary, so proceed with some caution. Add blueberries, sliced almonds, and some flax seed for added nutrition.

6. Cheese omelet with mushrooms, roasted peppers, and spinach: Eat it with a side of whole-wheat toast or an English muffin.

Each of these meals combines whole-grain fiber (e.g., toast, oatmeal, granola, and cereal) with a protein (e.g., eggs, yogurt, peanut butter, milk). Follow this pattern for a breakfast that will satiate you and hold you over until the next meal. Whatever you choose to eat for breakfast, make sure that you're not binging on it. So, control your portions and eat until you are full but not overfull.

Well-Balanced Lunch Ideas

So, half of your lunch should be fruit or veggies, one-third should be grains, and slightly less than one-fourth should be protein. There's so much variety here that it's hard to just limit it to a handful of recipes. With the ingredients explained, you can choose the items that work for you and create many different meals. Try to have at least three of the food groups covered in your lunch.

1. Fruit and veggies: For lunch, you could do a variety of sliced vegetables, or add them to a salad. You could even add them to a soup and get your veggies that way. For salads, try a mix of leafy greens, radishes, one-half an avocado, grape tomatoes, and carrots. Or go with one leafy green like spinach and add beets, carrots, cucumbers, and tomatoes to the salad. If salads aren't for you, experiment with sautéed vegetables like zucchini and mushrooms in soy sauce or roasted broccoli and peppers. Both options are great sides for grains and protein. If you would prefer a lunch that is more like a bunch of small sides than a full meal, choose two or three vegetables and slice them up for raw eating. When people think of food like this, they

think of carrots, tomatoes, and celery. But really, any vegetable will work so long as you're okay with eating them cold.

2. Grains: After you have your vegetables set up, you should add some grains. If you want a combination of grains and protein, try quinoa, barley, or buckwheat. If these are not things you're interested in, then have a side of potatoes or corn. You could even have toast or a sandwich with whole-grain bread and on the inside some meat, dairy, and vegetables. Savory oatmeal is also an option and is delicious with crumbled bacon, a poached egg, and spinach as a side.

3. Protein: Your lunch proteins can be ones that are easy to eat, like sliced meats, or meatballs, which are small enough to eat without a fork or knife. However, if you want to eat a variety, try some salmon filets, a beef stir-fry, roasted chicken breast, or tuna salad. If meat is not your thing, then try some braised tofu, roasted chickpeas, bean soup, or lentils. Eggs are also a good protein option.

4. Dairy: You can add a little bit of dairy to your lunch to have more flavor. Cheese is always a welcome ingredient to most foods. You could have a glass of milk with your lunch, too, or you could have a one-half cup of yogurt to wrap up your meal.

Here are some meal ideas:

- Mason jar salad with leafy greens, vegetables, quinoa, cheese, and dressing.
- Roasted chicken pieces and roasted potatoes, with a side of sliced peppers and tomatoes.

- Whole roasted sweet potato with beans, cheese, salsa, and corn. A side salad can round out this lunch if the potato alone isn't enough for you.

- Spinach and barley salad with grape tomatoes, poached eggs, feta cheese, and walnuts, plus a dressing of choice.

- Open-faced egg salad sandwich with whole-grain toast and a side salad.

- Bean soup, with a mix of several kinds of beans, cooked in bone broth or chicken broth. Some vegetables that work with soup are squash, celery, carrots, garlic, and onions cooked with the soup. You can also add some barley, egg noodles, or rice to the soup for your grain.

There is so much variety here. Find some recipes online that you're interested in and cook them for lunch. Just remember to include the right ratio of vegetables, fruits, grains, and proteins. The goal here is to not eat out for lunch every day. Mix it up. Choose foods, vegetables, and meats that are different so that you never get bored with your lunch. A key tip is to make your lunches on the weekend, store them in the fridge (or freezer), and then just bring them with you during your workday. Make sure that your lunch is going to keep you full and hold you over until your last meal of the day.

Well-Balanced Dinner Ideas

Dinner is obviously your last meal before your fast. If you're ending your eating window right before you go to bed, choose foods that are not going to keep you up at night. In this situation, stay away from heavily salted foods, heavy spices, or very fatty foods. These foods will disturb your sleep. If you have several hours between your last meal and bedtime, then feel free to eat things that will keep you full. Remember, the key strategy for feeling satiated is to mix protein and fiber. Meals that have these two things will keep you fuller for longer. You can repeat the ideas from the lunch area above, or you can branch out with heavier foods like stews and red meats. Here are some meal ideas:

- Whole-wheat spaghetti and turkey meatballs with tomato sauce, topped with some shredded Parmesan with a small side salad. You may add spinach to the tomato sauce.
- Salmon filet with asparagus, roasted tomatoes, and quinoa.
- Chicken curry with brown rice, spinach, and carrots.
- Bean chili with kidney, pinto, and black eye beans. Serve with whole wheat tortilla chips, cheese, and chives. The chili should have tomatoes and onions in it, but you can also add peppers, squash, or carrots to spruce it up.
- Tofu stir-fry with asparagus, bell peppers, onions, almonds, sesame seeds, and green beans. This can be served with brown rice or barley.

It's a good idea to have some variety with your dinner meals. Have some meatless meals during the week and add at least two meals with fish. This will provide you with some different nutrients and will also help so you don't get bored with your menu.

Cooking all these meals can feel really overwhelming if you're not into cooking. If you're interested, you can cook meals over the weekend and store them in the fridge or freezer. This will help ease your meal planning for the week. If you want to really try something different, you can use one of the meal deliveries services that provide you with either complete meals or the ingredients for the meals based on your nutritional requirements. These include companies like Blue Apron, Freshly, or Plated. These can be a good option if you don't know how to cook because they'll provide everything and give you step-by-step directions on how to make their products. Either way, you want to avoid eating out every day and try to skip the easy freezer meals unless they're packages of frozen vegetables. Ramen noodles are also not a well-balanced meal despite what your roommates at college taught you.

Chapter 3.
Benefits and risks of intermittent fasting

While reading this benefits and risks, keep in mind that not everyone will react the same way. How you react to fasting isn't going to be the same as how someone else does. So, look at your health with a critical eye and consider whether the benefits will help you or whether the risks will harm you. You can also just do a trial and error fast to see how your body will react, but always do so with wisdom.

It's important to mention some of the limitations of these studies. Intermittent fasting is so recent that there isn't enough research yet on the human experience while intermittent fasting. There is some research, but not a lot. More research has been done on animals that are like humans biologically, like some apes. Some less similar animals are rodents, and there are a lot of studies on fasting with rodents. Some of these will be mentioned here and some will be human studies. But all will help explain the benefits and risks.

Benefits of Intermittent Fasting

Generally intermittent fasting has way more benefits than risks. The one everyone knows about is weight loss. But there are so many other benefits too. One of the best benefits is how intermittent fasting changes your hormone levels, so that your insulin levels are lowered. There are also some other benefits for your heart, brain, and body.

Weight loss

Weight loss it the most well-known benefit of intermittent fasting. Even this book has the word "weight loss" in the title. During intermittent fasting, it's likely that you'll lose some weight. Whether you're following the easier 14/10 method or the harder alternate day method, you're going to lose some weight. There are a couple of reasons why this is, but the biggest one is because of calorie restriction.

Calorie restriction is one of the most common methods of weight loss recommended by doctors. In simplified 14/10 fasts and ones like it, you'll have some unplanned calorie restriction which can help you with weight loss. To get the most out of calorie restriction, you would want to follow the alternate day style of fasting. This is because there's just such a massive reduction in calories on those alternate days. Alternate day fasting has been found to be equivalent to regular, doctor approved, calorie reduction in multiple studies (Alhamdan et al., 2016; Klemple et al., 2010; Anson et al., 2003). Even better yet, because calorie reduction is interspersed with full regular meals every other day, this style of fasting is easier to stick with rather than a regular calorie restricted diet.

So, you can expect some weight loss while intermittent fasting. However, this also depends on other aspects of your lifestyle. We've talked about the importance of diet before, but we haven't talked about the importance of exercising. Doing regular exercising while intermittent fasting can also increase how much weight you lose, without losing a lot of muscle mass from the fast. You don't have to exercise heavily, but if you want to, you could go for a 30-minute walk, a bike ride or a swim. All of these can help maintain your weight loss while also maintaining your muscle mass.

The last thing to mention is that once you finish your fasting, in the case where you're not doing this for the rest of your life, you'll be less likely to regain the weight. Take it or leave it, but you'll still have some improvement in your weight with intermittent fasting.

Intermittent fasting can reduce insulin levels and insulin resistance. Did you know that one-third of Americans are diagnosed with pre-diabetes? That's quite a lot and is often due to our carb and sugar laden diets. So many people in the U.S. struggle with their blood sugar levels and insulin levels. Essentially, in prediabetes your blood sugar levels are consistently higher than normal, and your body tries to fix this by increasing your insulin. Insulin is what helps your body to absorb the glucose from your food to use as energy. However, when experiencing prediabetes, your cells become resistant to the insulin. This increases the cycle again, with more insulin coming into your bloodstream and more insulin resistance occurring. This can be very problematic and result in having a diagnosis of type 2 diabetes, stroke, obesity or heart disease. Intermittent fasting can help with your insulin levels and insulin resistance.

When intermittent fasting, the blood-glucose levels can be a little more controlled, insulin resistance is reduced, and insulin itself is also reduced. This is something that has been repeated in several studies. The insulin decreases because of the way the body uses the glucose from eating during the fasting period, but it also decreases because of weight loss that is also happening. In most studies, the type of fasting used to create some of the best changes in insulin levels was alternate day fasting. This makes a lot of sense, since it's also the style of fasting that results in the most weight loss.

Improved heart health is one of the benefits that needs to be better researched in humans. However, in animals intermittent fasting is very promising for improving heart health. Intermittent fasting helps improve cholesterol levels, blood pressure, and inflammation. All of which can lead to better heart health. Obviously, this is important because since there are so many things that can negatively affect heart health. So, if intermittent fasting can help reduce these things, then you'll have a lower risk of heart disease, heart attacks, and other cardiovascular problems.

There is some research that suggests intermittent fasting can help with ageing and brain health. It has to do with how your cells recuperate from cellular stress and metabolism. The research suggests that intermittent fasting can help reduce the likelihood of Alzheimer and Parkinson's diseases (Martin et al., 2009). While this research is very promising, there hasn't been enough human research to say this. However, the promise of better brain health is something to look forward to with intermittent fasting.

Risks of Intermittent Fasting

The risks of intermittent fasting are varied. However, for most people intermittent fasting isn't very risky. The risks you'll run into are bingeing, malnutrition, and difficulty with maintaining the fast. We've talked about bingeing quite extensively, so we're not going to discuss it much more. Suffice it to say, bingeing while you fast risks any of the benefits from fasting you might originally have. A bigger risk is malnutrition.

Malnutrition sounds alarming, but for the most part, you can prevent this by having well-balanced meals during your eating windows. The risk of malnutrition comes especially during the kinds of fast which include very low-calorie restriction on fasting days. Fasts like this are 5:2 fasts and alternate day fasting. If you're not eating the right nutrition throughout your week, the reduction in calories plus the poor nutrition can result in some of your dietary needs not being met. This could result in more weight loss, but also more muscle loss and other issues. To prevent this risk, you can ensure that your meals are nutritious and well-balanced. Have a variety of fruits and vegetables, try different meats and seafoods, and include grains unless you're following a specific diet like the keto diet.

Associated with malnutrition is dehydration. We get a lot of our daily water intake from the food we eat. But if you're eating a reduced amount of food during your day, or no food during your day, you're going to need to drink a lot more water than you normally do. If you're not keeping track of your hydration levels, it's possible for you to drink too little. To combat this risk, ensure that you're drinking enough by keeping a hydration journal. You could also track it in an app. Set up reminders to drink water and check your urine color. Light colored urine means good hydration, so check often despite how disgusting it might be to you.

Because fasting can be difficult to start, this can be one of the risks associated with it. You're going to feel hungry during the first couple weeks of following your fasting schedule. You may even feel uncomfortable, with mood swings, different bowel movements, and sleep disruptions. All of this can lead to you struggling with starting the fasts. They can also lead you to ignore greater warning signs that you shouldn't fast. These signs include changed heart rate, feelings of weakness, and extreme fatigue. These feelings shouldn't be ignored during the start. If you feel severely uncomfortable when you start your fast, you should stop and speak with your doctor.

Chapter 4.
All the different styles of intermittent fasting (16/8, 14/10, etc...)

Unlike other diets that are specific in the manner they're executed, intermittent fasting isn't a specific diet. There are a number of varied approaches to intermittent fasting that you can opt to execute depending on what works best for your needs and lifestyle. However, the principle is the same. Here are common ways to do intermittent fasting:

The 16/8 Method (Leangains Method)

This approach of intermittent fasting is also referred to as the Lean gains and is widely popular. Martin Berkhan, a fitness expert, came up with it. This approach of fasting involves 16 hours of a fast (fasting window) and 8 hours of eating (feasting window). When you follow this method, you can choose to skip breakfast or dinner depending on when you begin your 16 hours of fasting. For instance, when you have your last meal at 9 pm, you'll not eat again until 1 pm the next day when your feasting window begins. This essentially means you'll have to skip breakfast.

You can fit up to 3 meals into your feasting window. You can be strategic about your fasting and feasting windows while considering your lifestyle. For instance, if you're in a labor intensive job then you need to make sure your feasting window falls within the time when you'll be working. You can be entitled to taking coffee, tea, water, and other non-caloric drinks. Although intermittent fasting is not specific to the kind of food you should eat, it's advisable that you mostly focus on healthy eating.

> Implementing the 16/8 Approach

To following this intermittent fasting approach successfully, you'll need to keep track of everything you eat and do. Although this can be difficult in the beginning, it will get better with time. The reason for journaling is so that you stay focused and track results. You're at liberty to select your feasting and fasting windows even though the creator of this plan recommends the best time for the feasting to begin in the afternoon through to half-past eight because this is when you get to attend social activities. Additionally, you also get to cover the early hours of fasting while sleeping which is pretty much normal. Make sure you identify a time in your schedule when you can workout particularly after you've had your first or second meal during the feasting window. Once you're through with the exercise, have a large post-workout meal. You need ensure that you're consuming 60% of your total calorie intake post-workout. Ultimately, you shouldn't have more than three meals during the feasting window. The point is that you need to maintain a caloric deficit or simply eat at maintenance especially if your goal is to shed off excess weight and fat. When properly done, 16/8 will see you recompose your body so that you replace the fat with muscle.

Making 16/8 Work for You

Although it has been said to be the easiest of all the intermittent fasting approaches, following the 16/8 intermittent fasting approach is not easy. However, you can make it work for you by considering the following tips:

- Consume carbs on the days when you also get to work out so that you're able to burn the excess glucose.

- Incorporate sufficient amounts of proteins in your meals when the feeding window comes without attempting to compensate for low protein consumption where there was a shortfall.

- Avoid eating before your workout and instead, have a nutrient packed meal after your workout.

- You have to work out if you want to realize the results of following 16/8

- Aim at consuming food that is known to be nutritional powerhouses while shunning calorie bombs that offer little or no nutritional value. Ultimately, you shouldn't consume any calories during the fasting period.

You have the power to make the 16/8 intermittent fasting method to work for you. Make it fun and you will be amazed at the results you will achieve.

The Warrior Method

Ori Hofmekler, who is a fitness expert and former member of the Israeli Special Force, formulated the warrior approach. The idea was to imitate the diets of ancient warriors thus it involves consuming small portions of vegetables and fruits during the day and concluding a huge meal for dinner. This means that you're cycling lengthy periods of fasting and short eating windows. For instance, you can fast for 20 hours and only have 4 hours of feasting. This method recommends consuming certain vegetables and fruits while you're fasting. You can also take drinks with zero calories. Most importantly, these methods emphasize more on the quality of your diet.

The warrior method is far much strict compared to any other intermittent fasting approach. Interestingly, it is also the most effective in terms of achieving results and is not difficult to get started on it. This plan will mostly attract people with a tough personality because it is harsh in nature. I mean, how many people can be comfortable with having a single meal a day? On the downside, following the warrior method could also damage your relationship with food since it is mostly psychological.

➢ Implementing the Warrior Method

Before you dive into the warrior method, it's advisable that you calculate your BMR and determine the number of calories you'll need from carbs, fat, and proteins. A big portion of your consumption should be proteins, followed by carbs and then the rest of the calories. You should also set a time when you will be doing your workout keeping in mind the fasting window. You can only get into heavy workout in the feeding phase even this can be challenging because of how short the window is. Besides, since you're having one large meal you need ample time to eat and allow digestion to take place. Weigh your options and work out something reasonable. For instance, you can consider shortening the length of your workout so that you preserve your muscle mass and increase your fitness levels. Thus a High Intensity Interval Training (HIIT) becomes ideal because it pushes your heart rate up while giving you a long resting interval. You can repeat after 15 minutes and you're free to make any movement. Think about cycling, pushups, jump rope, sprinting and squats. The possibilities are endless.

Alternate Day Fasting

Just as the name suggests, with this approach you'll fast on alternate days. This is means that if you eat normally today then you'll fast for an entire day tomorrow and go to bed without food. You're only allowed to take water, unsweetened black tea and unsweetened black coffee that is calorie-free on the days when you're fasting. However, you could also opt to do a modified fast where you cap your calories on the day when you're fasting to 500. This means that you're limiting your normal intake by 25%.

> ➢ Implementing the Alternate Day Fast Approach

To succeed with the alternate day intermittent fasting approach, you should begin by clearly defining your eating and fasting window. This means that you identify the 12 hours of the day when you will be eating and the 36 hours during which to fast. For instance, if you have your first meals at 8 a.m. and the last at 8 p.m. on Monday, you can repeat this 4 times a week on Monday, Wednesday, Friday and Sunday. Fasting automatically begins after your last meal.

This approach has yielded results for so many people across the world because it contributes to losing weight and fat as well as boost your overall wellbeing. Following this intermittent fasting approach will give you up to 8% weight loss within the first 8 weeks. You will also have better cellular energy production along with enhanced insulin resistance. This intermittent fasting approach is considered to be the best if you are looking to induce autophagy. However, women must embrace this approach with caution as 36 hours of fasting can be a little too radical. In fact, women are advised to consider going for low-calorie intakes during the fasting window. A combination of alternate day fasting with strength training will enhance fat burning and better results.

➢ Pros of Alternate Day Fasting

Alternate day fasting offers a number of advantages that include:

- Extended lifespan and better metabolism.
- Easy to follow in the longtime hence can be adopted as part of your lifestyle.
- It can improve conditions such as asthma.
- It doesn't present the challenge of deprivation because you're free to eat anything within the feeding window.

Cons of Alternate Day Fasting

Some of the disadvantages that are linked to intermittent fasting are:

- You are likely to experience fatigue, dizziness, and hunger in the extreme during the first few days.
- This method doesn't emphasize the importance of exercise that plays an important role in fat burning

- This intermittent fasting approach is not recommended for people with a history of eating disorders.

Crescendo Fasting

Women are more sensitive to prolonged periods of fasting than men. As such, fasting results in hormonal imbalance that in effect leads to hunger, fatigue, mood swings and in some cases, weight gain. The crescendo approach to intermittent fasting is far much favorable for the female body because it's less demanding. This method doesn't require daily fasting instead, you fast for 2 or 3 alternate days in a week for 12 to 16 hours. This allows you to maintain a regular feeding plan on the non-fasting days. However, you must refrain from heavy workouts.

> ➢ Advantages of Crescendo Fasting

This approach to intermittent fasting has a number of advantages that include the following:

- This method of fasting is great for burning fat pockets hence slimming down without too much strain.
- Crescendo fasting is gentle on the female body hence it helps to maintain a hormonal balance that is important especially in women.
- Crescendo fasting is a great way to get yourself into intermittent fasting because if prepares you physically and mentally.

The Downside of Crescendo Fasting

Crescendo fasting could result in an irregular menstrual cycle. Should this happen to you then you must abandon the program immediately. You also need to keep in mind that this eating plan is not good for anyone who has had a bad relationship with food in terms of eating disorders.

- Eat Stop Eat (The 24 Hour Fast)

This intermittent fasting plan is the brainchild of Brad Pilon. It encourages fasting completely for at least one or two whole days a week (24hours to 48 hours). It doesn't have to be two consecutive days as long as you do a 48-hour fast within the seven days of the week. You are free to choose when you'll begin your fast. It can be from the time you have dinner to the following day same time. You're free to take water, coffee, and other drinks that don't contain calories when you're fasting to stay hydrated. This method can be difficult if you're new to intermittent fasting. As such, you may want to begin with other intermittent fasting protocols to get used to fasting.

- Spontaneous Meal Skipping

This intermittent fasting protocol is unstructured because you don't follow a prescribed eating plan. There are times when you're too busy or you simply don't feel like eating/hungry. You can practice spontaneous meal skipping when faced with such scenarios. This method is tied to the fact that the human body can survive extended periods of no food yet function optimally.

The 12/12 Intermittent Fasting Approach

This approach to intermittent fasting is considered to be the easiest to follow because it gives you an equal number of hours for fasting and eating. That is, you fast for 12 hours and eat for 12 hours. What makes this approach easy is that you can cover most of the fasting period in your sleep. However, you also must not have more than three meals during the feasting window. Going on a 12 hour fast allows your system to rest even as your insulin resistance is enhanced thus promoting weight loss. Don't panic if you experience a slight headache, nausea or uneasiness before your body gets used to this pattern of eating. This is simply a reaction to the withdrawal of sugar from your system. However, if you experience these symptoms in the extreme then stop fasting immediately. Remember, the body will begin to adjust gradually. Make sure you take lots of water as well as unsweetened beverages like coffee and tea.

Chapter 5.
How to step by step transition into each different style of intermittent fasting

The 5:2 Method

This is also called the "twice-a-week" method. While in the other protocol names, the numbers refer to hours, here the numbers refer to days. Essentially, the idea is that you will fast on two days out of seven and, on the other five days, you will eat normal while ensuring that your diet is healthy. On days on which you fast, you will want to limit your intake to 500 calories. This can be split in whichever way is suitable to you during the day.

This may be a good method to begin with as it does not involve any major changes and you can select the days of the week that are convenient for you to fast on. You can slowly increase or amend this protocol when you feel ready.

Alternate-Day Method

As the name suggests, this method involves fasting on every second day. For instance, on Monday you would fast and on Tuesday you would eat your normal healthy meals, on Wednesday you would fast again. On fasting days, it is ideal to reduce your calorie intake during meals to around 500 calories. There are methods that prescribe zero calories on fasting days, although this may not be the easiest option to start with. Once you are finding it easier to fast, you can certainly attempt a zero-calorie fast day.

Of course, you can choose any day to begin on, so your alternate days would differ from the example above depending on the day of the week that you start.

Time-Restricted Method

This is more of a traditional intermittent fasting method in which you restrict your eating time to specific hours within the day. Examples of this method would be the 16/8 technique or 14/10 technique. In these examples, we are now referring to hours with these numbers and not days.

With the 16/8 technique, you allow yourself an "eating window" of eight hours within the day. For the other 16 hours, you are fasting. It is imperative to demarcate these hours and have them be the same hours each day. This is a very popular technique as it is easier to work into your ordinary day. For instance, you may say that your eating window is from 11 a.m. to 8 p.m. Any meals you consume must be during this window of time.

The 14/10 technique works in exactly the same way as the 16/8 technique except you are allowing yourself a 10-hour eating window and a 14-hour fasting window.

You would then repeat this technique on as many or as few days during the week as you wish. You could choose to combine one of these methods with a day-based method; for instance, restrict yourself using the 16/8-hour protocol but combine it with the 5:2 protocol or the alternate-day method. You would then apply the 16:8 protocol on the days you select as per the day protocol.

This is a very good way to start easing yourself into the intermittent fasting lifestyle. It is, of course, very important to ensure that when you do eat, you are not binging and you are limiting your calories and making good choices about your meals.

The 24-Hour Method

This technique requires that you fast for 24 hours at a time. This could be from breakfast to breakfast or lunch to lunch. You could also select times of the day, for instance 13:00 on Tuesday to 13:00 on Wednesday.

This method is quite severe and difficult for beginners. You may experience side-effects such as dizziness, headaches, and lethargy. If you decide to try this method, it is not recommended that you do so more than once per week to begin with (Cleveland Clinic, 2019). Once you are further along in your intermittent fasting journey, you can increase 24-hour fasts to more than once a week if you wish.

Select and Commit

Now that you have decided which intermittent fasting method is best for you to use, it is important that you commit yourself fully to this method. As we did with our goals, use your journal to describe in the first person which method you are going to use, how you will go about using that method, and how you will expect to feel when you are using the method.

In your journal, near where you wrote down and described your goals, write, "I am committing myself to the (insert method name) technique of intermittent fasting."

Then go on to write as much as you can about the method, the days and times that you plan to use the method, and the feelings you expect to have while using the method. Visualization is a very important tool to use when you are embarking on any self-development journey. By preparing your mind for what is to come and experiencing the attainment of the goal before you have achieved it, you can mold your mind into a winning mindset, making any sacrifices you need to make along the way far easier.

It is important to select a method that will serve your goal. If you have set yourself a relatively steep weight loss goal, you may not attain that goal by only fasting two days per week. This does not necessarily mean that you should change the method you have selected, but perhaps you should adjust your goal by giving yourself a longer period to attain it. Either way, whether it is your goal or your method that you adjust, it is vital to ensure that both are in congruence with each other.

The most important thing, though, is starting. You can iron out the wrinkles in your schedule later when you do your first self-assessment. Don't allow yourself to be bogged down by the details or not start because you are overwhelmed by which protocol to choose. This is just your brain's way of delaying and, if you find yourself overthinking the various protocols, then you need to understand what lies beneath that overthinking. Usually it is going to be fear, perhaps a fear of failure and your brain is subconsciously implying that you can't fail if you don't begin. Well, we have news for your brain: by not beginning your intermittent fasting journey because you are afraid, you will not succeed; you are failing at the outset. There really is no failure in intermittent fasting. You will learn what works for you and what doesn't and how you can adjust things to work better. Just get started!

Chapter 6.
Intermittent fasting and calorie restriction

This is known as the principle of calorie restriction.

It is what Benjamin Franklin meant when he said, "To lengthen thy life, lessen thy meals."

This is an essential key to great longevity. It was a key to long life for Luigi Cornaro and it can be your key to long life as well. Calorie restriction, when it is of the nutrient-rich kind, has been verified many times in animal trials to where its effectiveness in extending life is almost universally accepted. In his book, The Art of Living Long, Cornaro had his own way of describing the virtues of caloric restriction. He said, "Whosoever wishes to eat much, must eat little." By this, he meant that eating less at each meal allows you to live longer, and you will end up having many more meals in the long run.

In Cornaro's case, eating less meant a daily regimen consisting of bread, vegetable soup with tomato, an egg, a little serving of meat, and about 14 ounces of fresh spring wine. (Wine that is made from the first pressing and with a low alcohol content). In all, he consumed a total of about 1500 calories per day.

But there is no need for your long life diet to be as limited in variety as his. Cornaro restricted his food choices to only those which fully agreed with him. He did not tolerate fruits very well, for example, and excluded all of those from his diet.

Your first step is to get an idea of how many calories you take in each day to maintain your normal weight. Then multiply that number by 80% or 90% to get the new calorie level you wish to achieve.

If your best estimate after keeping track is 2250 calories per day, for example, 80% of that would give you a calorie restriction target of 1800 calories per day.

For convenience when counting the calorie content of your foods, round off to the nearest five calories for each item.

Your daily total doesn't have to be exact, but you do want to get it correct to the nearest 50 calories or so.

Going by the 80% restriction rule, an 1800 calorie level may be just right for a 170 pound man to start achieving longevity results.

But a petite woman weighing only 105 pounds may actually gain weight eating this many calories. Her proper calorie intake may be only 1500 or so.

It is important that you not fall below your restricted calorie level on this plan. Losing weight very slowly is the key to achieving the longevity benefit you are seeking.

Note: If you are very slender already and your count shows you are eating less than 1800 calories per day, skip Rules #1 and 2, and go on to Rule #3.

If you don't want to figure your normal calorie intake, there is another approach that will also work.

Unless you are already very slender, try eating at the 1800 calorie per day level and see whether that is enough to induce a gradual weight loss of one to two pounds a month.

If not, adjust it down accordingly to perhaps 1600 or 1700. If 1800 calories causes you to lose more than 3 pounds the first month, adjust the level upward to 1900-2000.

Continue to adjust your calorie intake this way until you are achieving the steady loss of 1-2 pounds per month you need to reach your goal.

Rule #1: Maintain your caloric restriction until you slowly lose 10-12% of your normal or "set point" weight if you are a woman or 15-18% of your normal weight if you are a man.

Remember a time in your life when you were eating so that you weighed neither too much nor too little. Judge this by how good you looked and also by how that weight made you feel. Consider this as your "set point", or the weight your body naturally tries to defend and maintain.

If you are a woman, have as your calorie restriction target a body weight that is 10-12% less than that. A set point of 120 pounds would give you a goal of somewhere between 108 and 105. Exactly where you level out should be determined by where in that range you look and feel your best.

If you are a man, have as your goal a weight that is 15-18% less than your natural set point.

If you feel your normal weight is about 180, you would endeavor to come in at somewhere around 153 to 147, again depending on where you feel your best.

Ideally, it should take you at least six to nine months of calorie restriction to reach your new weight.

It is very important that you not try to rush this!

The Long Life "classic" foods plan is not meant as a crash diet. Even taking as long as a year or a year-and-a-half to arrive at your long life weight is perfectly okay and may actually be optimal in terms of effectively resetting your metabolism.

If you try to lose the weight too rapidly, your body may interpret this as the onset of starvation and drastically slow your metabolism as a survival measure.

Remember, you have the same "model" body that your cave-dwelling ancestor had 100,000 years ago, when environments were more difficult, and living conditions more unpredictable and harsh.

The energy conserving mechanism that helped your paleolithic ancestor survive a challenging winter is still present in your body today and can be triggered by any sudden drop in calorie intake.

So you don't want your body to think that you are running out of food, only that you are cutting back on your daily intake.

Rule #2: As much as possible, eat only "classic" or "near-classic" foods to make up your calorie total.

These are the foods our bodies were designed to thrive on with the most amount of nourishment per calorie, and the least amount of difficulty in processing metabolically.

Frozen fruits and vegetables without added ingredients are also acceptable. Organic whole grains and breads are also an excellent choice to include in your diet and strongly encouraged.

Main dishes should be prepared with healthy mono-saturated fats, such as olive or canola oil, and no added refined sugar. If you want to add a little extra sweetness to your entrees, a little frozen apple juice works well with many things or add some raw, unfiltered honey. The moderate use of spices and seasonings are also fine additions to enhance natural flavors.

Follow the advise of Luigi Cornaro, and choose only those nutrient-rich foods that fully agree with you. Avoid any that do not agree, no matter how healthy you might otherwise believe them to be.

Surprise: Some "Health Foods" Really Aren't

Examples of foods that are commonly thought of as health foods but aren't on the "classic" food list are tofu, energy bars, high-sugar granola, and most store-bought fruit juices that have had the fruit pulp removed or extra ingredients added like sugar or corn syrup.

Juicing that you do at home where you are throwing the whole fruit into the blender is fine. There you are only changing the consistency of the fruit and not removing any of the fiber or nutrients.

You may be surprised to see tofu listed here as a less than desirable food. It is, after all, a staple in many vegetarian diets.

Studies have implicated many processed soy products with a certain type of mental deterioration that occurs in middle-age if these are eaten for a long period of time.

Eating whole or sprouted soybeans is fine, however, as those are nutritionally complete and confer many health benefits in a long life diet.

Another Look at "The Staff of Life"

For bread, it is recommended that you select sprouted whole-grain breads. These breads are made from organic sprouted grains, and have a hearty texture and delicious taste you won't grow tired of.

Because they are composed of nutrient-dense sprouted grains, you may see these breads also referred to as flour-less breads.

These are more desirable than breads made from flour, because their vital nutrients haven't been lost or diminished through excessive milling or refining. Their main ingredients are sprouted grains, yeast, and sea salt.

You can find them in your health food store under the brand names Ezekiel or Essene. You may recognize these as biblical names and their recipes have in fact been passed down generation to generation through the centuries. You will also find recipes on the Internet if you like to make your own breads.

Sprouted breads freeze very well, so you can stock up with a half-dozen loaves or more when they go on sale.

Adding to the convenience is that these breads taste best when toasted, so they can go from your refrigerator straight into the toaster.

Refined flour is basically a "wrecked" food. The milling process destroys the structure of the grain kernel, causing the loss of many vital nutrients.

Most brands of refined flour bread also have undesirable added ingredients such as saturated oils, refined sweeteners, and chemical preservatives.

Eating a sour-dough bread occasionally or a whole wheat or whole rye bread made from a sour-dough starter won't harm you from a long life standpoint. They would be classified as "near-classic" foods. Those breads, although good for you, are not as optimal in nutrition as the sprouted breads.

What we are looking for is the most "bang per calorie" as far as great nutrition is concerned. In this regard, the sprouted breads that don't contain milled flour are distinctly better for you.

Living In Romania

If you lived on a farm in Romania, it would be a lot simpler to find and eat only naturally occurring "classic" foods.

In fact, those are the kinds of foods most people ate virtually everywhere in the world as recently as a hundred years ago, when heart disease and cancer were far less common than they are today.

In this ideal rustic environment today, you would be living in the equivalent of 19th century America with no pizza parlors or fast burger places in sight, and with an abundance of fresh harvested grains, wholesome meat and dairy products, and healthy fruits and vegetables as your main food staples.

Living in the modern industrialized world today, things are going to be more challenging, not because you can't find "classic" foods, but because there are so many tempting (and distinctly unhealthy) food choices distracting you and competing for the attention of your taste buds.

You will need to side-step that vast minefield of entertaining but health-depleting foods found virtually everywhere in society and seek out healthier alternatives that support your long life strategy and are still enjoyable to eat.

This does not mean you can never enjoy your favorite plate of spaghetti with meatballs and Parmesan cheese, or the warm bread and butter appetizer. Or the Spumoni ice cream afterward.

From a longevity standpoint, it's okay to have something like that on occasion. You will need to count it as part of your daily calorie total and maybe cut back on your food intake the next day to keep your average calorie intake on track.

The idea is that you should strive for 90-95% of your diet to be made up of foods from the "classic" categories.

Even if 5-10% of your calorie intake comes from conventional treats or less healthy food, you can still reach your long life potential. The trick is limiting the unhealthy food choices to a small part of your overall diet.

Preventing the "Sugar Blues"

At the head of a list of foods that should be avoided whenever possible are refined sweeteners in all their forms. These seemingly harmless substances should be avoided like Grandma's belladonna, even though many of us find creative ways to give in to temptation more often than we should. The subtle and numerous ways in which processed sugar assists in undermining our health makes for a major discussion in itself.

Create Your Own Long Life Menu

With the Long Life "classic" foods diet, you are free to make up any meals you like, using the foods that appeal to you the most. The only guidelines are that most of the food choices you include should be of the "classic" or "near-classic" type.

Don't eat something your body is not happy with just because you think it might be healthy for you. This important point was something Luigi Cornaro emphasized in his discourses on long life.

Rule #3: Once you have gradually reached your new "long life" weight through nutrient-dense calorie

restriction, level off at that weight by slowly increasing your caloric intake by 100-200 calories per day more than before.

This will cause you to stop losing the 1-2 pounds per month you had been steadily losing, and bring you in for a "soft landing" at your desired weight.

If you find yourself starting to gain back some of the weight you have lost, reduce your calorie intake again until your weight levels off.

Once you have engineered the "soft landing" at your new Long Life ideal weight, it is time for you to fully appreciate your more energetic, healthier, and more youthful looking body.

Chapter 7.
The right motivation and mindset to stick with your plan

To achieve your weight loss and fitness goals, it is quintessential that you stick to the diet for at least a month to see any positive changes. If you want to stick to this diet, then you need to be self-motivated. There will be days when you don't have the motivation to keep going.

Set Your Goals

Before you decide to start a diet, it is time to analyze why you want to start a diet. What are the reasons why you wish to diet? What are your goals? You might want to lose weight, improve your fitness levels, or even lead a healthier life. Reasons tend to vary from one individual to another. If you don't set any goals for yourself, you will quickly lose motivation after a couple of weeks of dieting. However, while setting goals. There are a couple of simple things you must keep in mind. Ensure that the goals you set are specific, measurable, attainable, relevant, and time bound. Even if one of these ingredients is missing, then the chances of attaining such a goal will reduce.

If you set any unrealistic goals for yourself, you are setting yourself up for failure. For instance, a goal like, "I want to lose 40 pounds within four weeks," is quite unrealistic. By setting such lofty goals, you are setting yourself up for failure. When you cannot attain such an impossible goal, you will be demotivated, and you will quickly lose interest in dieting altogether. Any goal that you set needs to have a time limit. If you don't set a time limit for yourself, procrastination can creep in, and the likelihood of sticking to the diet will also reduce. Therefore, an ideal goal would be, "I want to lose two to three pounds every month."

Pick a date

You must always pick a date to start this diet. Don't be in a hurry and think that you can get started with this diet right away. There are a couple of things you need to do before you can begin to diet. For instance, you will need to stock up on all the ingredients you require to cook keto-friendly meals. Apart from this, you will also need to prepare yourself mentally to get started with the new diet. All this takes planning and preparation. You cannot skip these two necessary steps if you want to stick to the diet in the long run. When you opt for a specific date, ensure that you start dieting, from that day itself. Don't procrastinate, and don't tell yourself that you can start dieting from tomorrow. That "tomorrow" might never have come around. Maybe you can mark the date on your calendar to remind yourself that you are supposed to start with your diet.

Meal Plan

To ensure that you stick to the diet, you will need a meal plan. The good news is you don't have to create a meal plan for yourself. There is a detailed meal plan in this book. You can use it to get started with your new diet. Ensure that you include plenty of variety. Whenever you plan, the meals out for a week. If the food you eat starts getting repetitive, you will quickly lose interest to stick to your diet. Also, when you have a meal plan in place, it becomes easier to shop for groceries. If you know that you have a healthy meal waiting for you at home, the temptation of eating out will also reduce.

Make Calories Count

A common reason why a lot of people lose interest in dieting is because of hunger pangs. Ensure that you make every calorie count. Don't binge on unhealthy foods and instead, opt for nutrient-dense options. When your tummy is full, the urge to snack on junk food will reduce. If your daily calorie intake is 1800 calories, then ensure that you manage to eat at least two well-balanced, hearty meals. You can undoubtedly blow this calorie count by binging on a pint of ice cream, but it will do you no good.

Grocery Shopping

It is time to clean your pantry! Raid your kitchen and discard any unhealthy foods you find. Get rid of all cookies, cakes, chocolates, sodas, and other foods you must not eat while on the keto diet. Out of sight and out of mind is the best policy when it comes to dieting. If temptations surround you, the urge to give in will increase. Instead, stock up your pantry will keto-friendly ingredients. Once you have all the ingredients you need, it becomes easier to cook as well. Always prepare a grocery list before you go shopping and stick to this list.

Visualization

Whenever you are running low on motivation, remind yourself of the reasons why you started dieting. Think about the goals you want to attain. Start visualizing your goals. Think about how wonderful and happy you will feel when you attain your goals. While doing this, also think about how disappointed you would be if you didn't attain those same goals. While visualizing your goals, try to make the visualization as detailed as you possibly can. If you want, you can create a visualization board for yourself. Take a sheet of paper, make a note of your goal on it, and place it somewhere visible. Glance at it daily. It will act as a subconscious reminder for your mind. Fill this board up with positive affirmations, quotes, or even images that motivate you to stick to the diet.

A Dieting Buddy

The best way to ensure that you stay on track and stick to your diet is to find a dieting partner for yourself. Maybe you can start this diet with your partner, a friend, a loved one, family member, or anyone else. If you want, there are plenty of online forums; you can join and interact with others who are going through the same situation that you are in. When you do this, you will realize that you aren't alone. This, by itself, will give you plenty of motivation to keep going.

Chapter 8.
What to eat and what not to eat

Because you are reducing the number of calories that you consume, it is important that you ensure that every calorie that goes into your body counts. This is why you need to go for only foods that have a high nutrient quantity. Foods that are rich in fiber would also help to make you feel full.

- Herbs and spices
- Lean proteins
- Whole grains
- Vegetables
- Fruits
- Low or no-fat dairy products

Fruits and Vegetables

These are the perfect choice for the low-calorie diet as they offer you less of what you do not want which is the fat and calories while supplying you with more of what your body needs; fiber and nutrients.

Low-Fat Dairy and Lean Proteins

Sources of lean protein include grilled fish, chicken, and low-fat dairy products. They remove the extra calories in fat and still give you the protein that your body needs.

Whole Grains

You cannot totally make away with carbohydrates as your body needs them. But you have to go for the right one which is the whole grains that would supply more nutrients to your body along with your calories.

Herbs and Spices

These add flavor to your food without adding calories and fat. However, it is important that you watch your intake of sodium.

Foods to Reduce

- Sweetened beverages
- Rich, fatty foods (excess intake)
- Refined carbohydrates (excess intake)

Rich, Fatty Foods (in Excess)

While it is not advisable to totally leave out these foods from your menu, you would need to ensure that they do not make up most of your daily calorie intake as you may end up regretting the decision. These foods include butter, fatty cuts of meat, oil, cheese, and sugar. They contain lots of calories and would fill up your required calorie intake faster without achieving the desired results. This also applies to sweetened beverages. You can make use of non-nutritive or artificial sweeteners to reduce your calorie intake but it is better that you concentrate more on good foods rather than sugar-free junk foods. That said, you can still treat yourself to 100 to 150 calories daily be it chips, candies, or any other sweet treat. Just be conscious of the portions so that you do not eat more than you should. You can also go for healthier treats like a small glass of red wine or dark chocolate rather than purely junk foods. The antioxidants contained in the 2 examples may be good for your body.

Refined Carbohydrates (in Excess)

There are no foods that you should totally remove from your diet in the low-calorie diet. But it is important not to fill up your daily calorie quantity from simple carbs while missing out on important nutrients. These carbs would also make you feel hungry faster.

1,200-Calorie Diet Meal Plan

To start your menu plan, you would need to select foods that are low in calories and high in fiber like vegetables and fruits, low-fat protein sources and whole grains. Below, I have included two 1,200 calories daily menu to help you get started. The first is a 1,215-calorie menu that does not have any non-nutritive sweeteners added to it.

Breakfast

- Oatmeal – 1 cup
- Honey – 1 tablespoon
- Non-fat milk – ½ cup
- Plain tea or coffee as a beverage – 1 cup
- Blueberries – ½ cup

Lunch

- Water as a beverage

- 100% whole grain bread – 2 slices, tomato slice, deli-sliced turkey breast, mustard, and lettuce – 1 tablespoon
- Sliced carrots – ½ cup

Dinner

- Water with a slice of lemon
- Green beans – 1 cup
- Baked salmon – 3-ounces
- Salad with raw spinach – 1 cup, broccoli florets – ½ cup and cherry tomatoes - 5. Use lemon juice for dressing

Snacks

- Strawberries – 1 cup
- Several cups of water
- One apple with 12 almonds
- Plain yogurt - ½ cup with honey – 1 tablespoon
- Non-fat milk – 1 cup

Nutritional Information

- Total calories: 1,215
- Fiber: 28 grams
- Total Fat: 17.7%
- Total Carbohydrates: 59.3%
- Total Protein: 23%
- Sodium: 1,402 milligrams
- Cholesterol: 94 milligrams

- Sugar: 107 grams
- Saturated Fat: 5 grams

This second meal plan is a 1,218-calorie menu that does not have any non-nutritive sweeteners added to it.

Breakfast

- Whole-grain corn cereal – 1 cup
- Non-fat milk – ½ cup
- Sucralose – 1 packet
- 100% orange juice – 1 cup

Lunch

- Diet soda
- Salad made up of a one-half cup of cherry tomatoes, two ounces of albacore tuna (packed in water, two cups of field greens, and two tablespoons of balsamic vinegar as a dressing.

Dinner

- White wine – 1 Small glass
- Baked sweet potato – 1
- 3-ounce pork chop – 1
- Asparagus (steamed) – 1 cup
- Olive oil – 1 tablespoon

Snacks

- Lots of water with lemon or lime slices
- Pita bread – 1 small, and two tablespoons of hummus – 2 tablespoons
- Low-fat, sugar-free fruit-flavored yogurt – 1 serving
- One pear
- Baby carrots – 2/3 cup, with fat-free vegetable dip – 1 ounce
- Blueberries – 1 cup

Nutrition Information

- Total Calories: 1,218
- Fiber: 24 grams
- Total Fat: 14.6%
- Total Carbohydrates: 56.8%
- Total Protein: 22.6%
- Sodium: 1,615 milligrams
- Cholesterol: 116 milligrams
- Sugar: 86 grams
- Saturated Fat: 5.0 grams

1,500-Calorie Diet Meal Plan

To achieve a calorie intake of 1,500 every day, your DRI should have the following:

Note: DRI stands for Dietary Reference Intake

- Fiber: between 28 - 33.6 grams
- Total Carbohydrates: 130 grams

- Total fat: between 33 - 58 grams

- Sodium: 2,300 mg

- Total Protein: between 46 - 56 grams

- Cholesterol: Maximum of 200 – 300 grams

- Sugar: Maximum of 20 to 36 grams

- Saturated Fat: Maximum of 15 grams

Based on the parameters above, your menu would slightly vary depending on if you are watching your sugar intake or not. Below, you would see sample menus to guide you in creating yours.

Menu 1

Breakfast

- Whole-grain toast – 1 slice, with almond butter – 1 tablespoon
- Orange – 1
- Hardboiled egg – 1
- Plain coffee or tea – 1 cup

Lunch

- Sliced of carrots – ½ cup
- Whole-grain bread – 2 slices, Swiss cheese – 1 slice, Roast beef – two-ounce sliced, and mustard – 1 tablespoon
- Nonfat milk as a beverage – 1 cup

Dinner

- White wine – 1 small glass

- Chicken breast fillet – 1 3-ounce, with Salsa – 2 tablespoons

- Cooked black beans – ½ cup

- Cooked broccoli with lemon juice – 1 cup

- Whole-wheat dinner roll – 1, with butter – 1 teaspoon

Snacks

- Lots of water

- One nectarine – 1

- Blueberries ½ cup

- Sweetened grapefruit juice – 1 cup

- Plain yogurt – ¾ cup, with honey – 1 tablespoon

- Pecan halves – 10

Nutrition Information

- Total Calories: 1,498

- Fiber: 32 grams

- Total Fat: 20.5% (35 grams)

- Total Carbohydrates: 51.7% (201 grams)

- Total Protein: 23% (89 grams)

- Sodium: 1,934 milligrams

- Cholesterol: 295 mg

- Sugar: 87 grams

- Saturated Fat: 6 grams

Menu 2

This particular menu is for people that need to watch their intake of sugar, like people with prediabetes and diabetes. Rather than using sugar, you can make use of non-nutritive sweeteners.

Breakfast

- Cooked oatmeal – 1 cup, with walnuts – ½ ounces
- Grapefruit – ½
- Nonfat milk – 1 cup
- Stevia sweetener or sucralose – 1 or 2 packets

Lunch

- Baked salmon (no oil) – 3 ounces
- A salad with spinach – 1 cup, cherry tomatoes – ½ cup, feta – 1 ounce, and balsamic vinegar (no oil) – 2 tablespoons
- Diet soda – 1

Dinner

- Peeled shrimp - 6-ounces, add diced green pepper – 1 small size, sautéed in a tablespoon of garlic and olive oil
- 100% whole-grain dinner roll – 1 small
- Cooked brown rice – 1 cup
- Water with a slice of lime or lemon

Snacks

- Apple – 1
- Air-popped popcorn (butter-less) – 2 cups

- One serving sugar-free, low-fat, fruit-flavored yogurt

- Raw baby carrots – 2/3 cup, with one ounce of fat-free dip

- Strawberries – 1 cup

- Lots of water with slices of lime or lemon

Nutrition Information

- Total Calories: 1,496

- Fiber: 25 grams

- Total Fat: 22.4% (37 grams)

- Total Carbohydrates: 51.3% (193 grams)

- Total Protein: 26.4% (99 grams)

- Sodium: 1,496 mg

- Cholesterol: 428 milligrams

- Sugar: 49 grams

- Saturated Fat: 11 grams

After you have inputted all the required details into the weight loss calculator, the calculator would present you with a daily calorie goal. This goal contains the required number of calories you need to consume daily to be able to get to your weight loss goal within the timeframe you selected. For weight loss purposes, you would get a calorie deficit factored into the final number while calorie surplus is included in the final number for weight gain.

Several people think that cardio training is just to take long but boring jogs on the treadmill or even pedaling an upright bike for an extended time. However, cardio training is all about high-intensity interval training (HIIT), which interchanges between the very high-intensity exercise rounds and either a complete rest or a low-intensity round of exercise. This is different from the 30 to 60 minutes of ongoing steady-state cardio that the majority do on the cardio machines. HIIT workouts are done in lesser time than the old cardio workout but achieve the same if not better results. Benefits of doing the HIIT workouts are:

- It raises your metabolic rate to help burn extra calories while exercising and resting.

- It increases the anaerobic and aerobic pathways that help to utilize and take in more oxygen during steady-state training. It also helps you carry out the anaerobic exercises for a longer time.

- It helps you to break through training tables.

Increase in EPOC (excess post-exercise oxygen consumption) which leads to a longer and higher burning of calories even after you have stopped the exercise.

Chapter 9.
What to drink

A lot of people drink coffee. Coffee itself has become a sort of lifestyle commodity. Coffee comes in so many forms, styles, and even flavors. Most people do have a daily routine that includes coffee of some kind.

Coffee

When considering coffee and your 16/8 intermittent fasting method, during your eating window, coffee with milk and sweeteners is fair game! Remember that any additives have calories and carbohydrates, so moderation is key.

What about during the fasting cycle? Well, coffee can still be consumed, but without any additives. Some people can't handle the harshness of black coffee and may not want to try this.

There are many different coffee roasts available on the market now. Some are even flavored! When looking into the health benefits of coffee that will complement the 16/8 intermittent fasting plan, let's take a closer look at Dark Roast Coffee.

What is dark roast coffee?

Dark roast coffee is often described as coffee with a full, intense flavor that can be bittersweet, bold, and even smoky. Essentially, dark roast coffee beans are roasted to an internal temperature that is about 50-

100 degrees F higher than light roast beans. The higher temperatures change the composition of the sugars, caffeine, and flavor of the beans.

Often times, dark roast coffee can be easier going down black than light roast, which means it is an excellent no calorie beverage during fasting periods.

A dark roast tends to have a little less caffeine than a light roast, but anything with caffeine should be drunk before or during your eating window.

Dark roast coffees have also shown greater health benefits than light roast coffee. First off, some people with sensitive gastrointestinal tracts that can't drink coffee easily have found that they can drink black dark roast coffee with little to no irritation.

Research has been done into Molecular Food and Nutrition that has indicated dark roast coffee can restore Vitamin E, red blood cells, and glutathione much more effectively than the average light roast coffee. Further research in that study showed that dark roast coffee showed a decrease in body weight in pre-obese individuals.

Wow! Who knew that dark roast coffee could assist in weight loss? That sounds even better when we are talking about beverages that can be drunk during a fasting period on an intermittent fasting plan designed for weight loss!

While any black coffee is acceptable to drink during your fasting cycle, the dark roast has some better health benefits that actually align with a weight loss goal!

Tea

Some people just aren't coffee drinkers. There is nothing wrong with that! There are other options, such as tea. Tea is another readily available beverage that is very low calorie when consumed with no additives.

Just like coffee, tea can come in so many forms and styles with different flavors, serving methods, and dressings.

Tea with no additives is an approved fasting period beverage because it is low calorie, and most tears are also low carb unless they are fruit-based flavors.

There is one tea type that is right in line with some superfoods and has extraordinary benefits on the body and mind. It used to be a secret but has slowly been gaining more attention. This particular tea is absolutely perfect to work alongside your 16/8 intermittent fasting method!

Green Tea. Most everyone has heard of green tea in one form or another, such as macha, or a green tea Frappuccino, or as a flavor in ice cream even!

We are talking about just plain old loose leaf or in a bag green tea! It is quite literally one of the healthiest beverages on the planet. Whether you drink it warm in a mug or have it iced, the benefits of green tea are huge! And, not surprisingly, go hand in hand with many of the benefits and goals of the 16/8 intermittent fasting method!

Some of the health benefits of green tea include:

- Improved brain function
- Increase fat burning
- Improved physical performance
- Decreases risk of infection
- Reduces the risk of type 2 Diabetes
- Lowers cardiovascular disease risk
- Help weight loss
- Prevent obesity
- Increase longevity

So what is it about green tea that makes it so healthy?

First of all, green tea is packed full of nutrients in the form of bioactive compounds. One of the most prominent compounds in green tea is ECGC, or Epigallocatechin Gallate, which has been studied extensively as a treatment for various diseases. Green tea also contains antioxidants and minerals beneficial to good health.

Green tea contains caffeine. Lower levels than coffee, but still enough to stimulate the brain. Between the caffeine and amino acid in green tea called L-theanine green tea actually assists in brain function. It increases dopamine, has an anti-anxiety effect, and increasing the alpha waves in the brain.

The caffeine and L-theanine work together synergistically to overall improve brain function.

These brain benefits aren't just for short term; they can extend to long term brain protection from neurodegenerative diseases.

Most weight loss supplements include green tea. That is because green tea has been proven in human trials to increase the metabolic rate and induce fat burning at a faster rate.

With an increased metabolic rate, fat is burned quicker. Not to mention, green tea-induced weight loss has also been known to target the abdominal fat stores, reducing belly fat and waist circumference.

The antioxidants in green tea have been known to reduce the risks of breast cancer, prostate cancer, and colorectal cancer. Green tea drinkers are 20 to 30 percent less likely to develop breast cancer, 48 percent less likely to develop prostate cancer, and 42 percent less likely to develop colorectal cancer. Those are pretty big odds!

The catechins that are contained in green tea have multiple biological effects within the body. Influenza is a nasty virus and somewhat common. Green tea catechins can actually inhibit the development of influenza viruses, and others, which also reduces the risk of infection.

Then there is something as common as mutant strains of Streptococcus which contribute to oral bacteria, plaque, tooth decay, and gum infection. Guess what can fight and reduce the growth of mutant Streptococcus? Yup! Green tea! That means green tea can even combat bad breath.

Green tea has the effect of lowering blood sugar levels in the body. Green tea drinkers are 18 percent to 42 percent less likely to develop type 2 diabetes. Whether or not green tea can help reduce the use of diabetic medication was not part of that particular study. It may be more functional as a preventative.

Cardiovascular disease is often caused when LDL cholesterol and triglycerides are oxidized. Green tea helps reduce oxidation levels. Green tea drinkers are known to have 31 percent less of a chance to develop potentially life-threatening cardiovascular disease. Since cardiovascular disease is one of the most common killers today, that is a huge benefit!

Since green tea can reduce cardiovascular disease and cancer risks, it has been known to increase longevity for the body. As a whole, green tea has also been known to decrease the mortality rate for any cause by 23 percent in women and 12 percent in men.

This is absolutely amazing information. To have a beverage that can be consumed during fasting periods and your designated eating window that provides similar and different benefits to your 16/8 intermittent fasting plan is incredible.

Of course, green tea isn't a cure-all, but it certainly does give other low calorie and low carbohydrate drinks a run for their money in the health department!

How do you make the perfect cup of green tea? Many people shy away from green tea because it can have a bitter taste or a strong aftertaste. Fortunately, there is a way to brew the perfect cup of green tea.

First, you want to make sure you have the right amount of tea. A standard tea bag is fine for an average sized mug. If you are using loose leaf tea, about one teaspoon of the tea leaves per six ounces of water is a good ratio.

The water should be fresh and cool, tap, spring, or filtered. Distilled water isn't ideal for tea as it can provide a flat flavor.

For green tea, you want to bring the water just short of boiling, roughly 160 degrees to 180 degrees F.

In a mug, you should have your tea bag or loose-leaf tea in an infuser. Pour the hot water over the tea and cover with a plate. Allow the tea too steep for one to three minutes. Depending on how strong you like your tea, you might want to taste it in thirty-second intervals to avoid brewing.

Once brewed to the desired flavor, uncover and take the teabag or infuser out. There is your perfect cup of green tea. During your eating window, sweeten with a little milk and/or honey if you like.

Of course, there are hundreds of varieties of tea. Black tea, white tea, herbal tea, oolong tea, green tea, twig tea, and then each of those is broken down into several other categories of tea like Earl Grey, Irish Breakfast, Darjeeling, and different flavors too.

Tea is a great low-calorie beverage in any form or flavor. If you are looking to maximize your health and weight loss benefits with a beverage that keeps on giving during your fasting period, green tea is a great option!

Decaf vs. Caffeine

Most coffees and teas come with decaf and caffeinated options. Generally, people like to drink their caffeine in the morning or afternoon to help wake them up or give them a second wind to get through the day.

With a 16/8 intermittent fasting plan, it is recommended that you drink any caffeinated beverages in the morning or at the beginning of your eating window. Decaf beverages should be consumed when you're eating window closes.

There are a few reasons for this. First off, if you have your fasting schedule set up so that you will sleep through a portion of your fasting cycle, then caffeine has the potential to keep you awake longer. If the goal is to sleep through most of your fasting cycle, try not to tempt fate by drinking beverages that could keep you up.

Additionally, caffeine stimulates the mind and body. If you are in a stimulated zone, your body will be more sensitive, and you can start feeling more intensely hungry.

If you don't like decaf beverages, sticking to water once you're eating window closes is a good plan. If you don't like caffeinated beverages, then you don't really need to worry.

There are some different benefits for decaf and caffeinated beverages, though.

Let's look at what caffeine has to offer in terms of benefits first. Well, it can stimulate the metabolic process to encourage fat burning. However, this is usually a temporary effect, and once your body is used to caffeine, it stops responding to the metabolic stimulation and the benefit goes away.

Some other benefits of caffeinated beverages include:

- Improved mood

- Better reaction time

- Increased memory and mental function

- Enhanced athletic performance

- Reduce depression

- Reduced risk of cirrhosis of the liver

Many of these benefits, such as mood, brain function and memory, and athletic performance, are going to be based on the body's tolerance of caffeine. If you drink caffeine every day, your body will most likely be acclimated to the presence of caffeine, and the benefits won't be as prominent or long term.

Caffeine is a stimulant that can and does reduce tiredness, increases alertness, and increases energy levels. However, caffeine is a substance that stimulates parts of the brain and body to feel less tired and more alert. It doesn't actually provide the body and mind with energy sources or better neural pathways.

Drinking caffeine can contribute to insomnia, especially if drunk closer to your designated sleep time. If consumed regularly and in large quantities, if you miss a day or stop drinking caffeine, your body will feel sluggish, and you'll have headaches. This is essentially your body 'coming down' to its natural levels of energy and alertness. Consumption of caffeine is recommended in moderation.

What about decaffeinated beverages? Well, they kind of have a bad reputation, unfortunately. Beverages such as herbal tea, which are innately decaf, are often naturally sweet, flavorful, and enjoyable.

Decaf coffee is the culprit when it comes to the negative stigma. However, it is an undeserved reputation because decaf coffee definitely has benefits. Some might even be more desirable than caffeinated coffee benefits.

While decaf coffee isn't one hundred percent caffeine free, it is drastically lower in caffeine than regular coffee. However, decaf coffee is loaded with nutrients and antioxidants that benefit overall health.

Decaf coffee benefits include:

- Decreased risk of Type 2 Diabetes
- Reduced risk of premature death
- Reduction in acid reflux and heartburn

The above examples have been studied with both regular coffee and decaf coffee. The general scientific consensus is that decaf is better at reducing acid reflux and heartburn than regular coffee. Decaffeinated coffee drinkers have also shown a higher decrease in the development of Type 2 diabetes than regular coffee drinkers.

Premature death is a pretty vague and broad term. However, decaffeinated coffee has shown decreases in unexpected premature death with its drinkers, more so than regular coffee.

Alright, so both caffeinated and decaffeinated coffees and teas have benefits. Remember that when following the 16/8 intermittent fasting method, try to drink caffeinated beverages before or during your eating window. Reserve decaffeinated beverages for after your eating window.

Water

This is obviously the most readily available and healthy drink when fasting. Taking water will ensure that you maintain a healthy system in addition to aiding the absorption of nutrients. Water also contains minerals that play an important role in the restoration of your body's electrolyte and mineral balance. When you fast, you lose a reasonable volume of electrolytes as well as the fluid that is also beneficial for better joint and muscle support. The water can either be plain, flavored or carbonated as long as it's calorie free.

Apple cider vinegar

Diluting apple cider vinegar in water and taking it will not break your fast. According to a 2018 study, apple cider vinegar has properties that promote positive metabolic processes that help in shedding off weight. In fact, daily consumption of apple cider vinegar will result in reduced amounts of the overall bad cholesterol in the body.

Chapter 10.
Intermittent fasting and autophagy

The weight-loss world has shifted from diet charts to fasting for long hours. Staying hungry for a long time is a great way to lose weight. This technique is called 'intermittent fasting'. And it works on the principle of autophagy.

Auto- self

Phage- eat

The word autophagy means when something eats itself. And that is exactly what triggers the reduction of body mass in humans. Your body stays in the growth mode when you eat regularly. It generates energy to do work by using food molecules. The cells store the extra energy inside them in the form of fat. The waste products that enter the cells in the body (due to internal and external factors) gather inside them. This affects your organs, tissues, and eventually, your health and weight too.

But when you stop eating and start fasting, your body starts looking for sources of energy. As a result, the fat stored in the cells is broken down, and energy is released from them. Therefore, autophagy is a process where the body cells destroy their damaged parts and proteins and then recycle them in order to build themselves.

You can also view autophagy as a process where the cells in the body burn away the toxins stored in them and then use the remains to make something new. Many tissues and organs start the process of autophagy when they are deprived of food.

But How Does Your Body Know When To Start The Process Of Autophagy?

A signal must be sent to the organs to start breaking down the cells to produce energy. This can be done in many ways. It is not just fasting that can start autophagy in your body. Here are some other ways of losing weight that you can opt for.

Exercise

The more stress you create in the muscles and cells of your body, the more strongly the cellular cleanup phase will be triggered. All the extensive forms of exercise, including jogging, sprinting, weight training and physical training, regulate autophagy by inducing stress in the body. When the body is highly worked up, it needs energy that it gains by burning up the cellular waste.

Cold Showers

Yes, cold showers can also invoke healthy autophagy inside you. Studies have shown that people who swim during the winter exhibit higher levels of cell repair and recycling. Therefore, taking cold showers regularly can help you lose weight and stay healthy.

Steam Bath

Subjecting yourself to high temperatures through saunas and steam baths generates heat stress inside you. This heat results in the destruction and recycling of cancerous as well as damaged cells.

A trip to a spa can be good for relaxing, rejuvenating, losing weight and staying preventing diseases. Besides, exposing yourself to strong heat also helps to cure depression by naturally releasing heat shock proteins.

Intermittent Fasting

There are indicators in your body that activate or cease certain processes. The hormonal levels are one of them. When you begin intermittent fasting, you deprive the cells of essential nutrients. This activates the hormone glucagon in the body. This hormone works in opposition to insulin. While insulin increases blood sugar levels, glucagon brings them down to maintain the balance. The two hormones are like the ends of a see-saw.

When you are fasting, insulin levels go down, and, as a result, glucagon levels go up. This rise triggers autophagy. Your body gets the message that it is time to break down the stored fats in the body cells increase the insulin levels again.

Antioxidants

Though antioxidants do not directly invoke the process of autophagy in your body, they have been known to indirectly work towards it.

Foods rich in antioxidants support the process when you are fasting, which in turn ensures that you undergo a healthy and balanced autophagy process.

Is There Something That Can Stop Autophagy?

There are factors that can stop your autophagy process. The major one is the mTOR. It stops the autophagy in your body when there are enough nutrients in the cells. It is highly sensitive and eating as little as 50 calories can increase the level of mTOR.

If you consume fats, it might not raise your insulin levels, and it might keep the mTOR levels suppressed. But high amounts of ketones and fats would break your fast.

Here is a list of things that you can take to keep your insulin levels low and let your body continue the waste removal process of your cells.

- Green Tea
- Coconut Oil
- MCT Oil
- Ginger compounds
- Galangal
- Reishi mushroom extracts
- Black coffee
- Apple cider vinegar

All these items can help to boost autophagy in your body.

Is It Just For Weight Loss?

Absolutely not. When the cells renew themselves by burning up the waste inside them, they do more than decrease your weight. Clean and healthy cells decrease the risk of developing diseases. Many forms of cancer, neurodegenerative diseases like Alzheimer's and Parkinson's, and metabolic and autoimmune diseases can be prevented through autophagy.

It helps fight infectious diseases and regulates inflammation. It has also been associated with fighting depression and schizophrenia. Fasting-induced autophagy is very helpful in keeping you healthy and preventing medical conditions. It is always good to get rid of the waste around and inside you. A clean environment is healthy and keeps you from getting sick.

Here is a list of major benefits of autophagy, both inside and outside of a body cell.

- Increases metabolism
- Decreases oxidative stress
- Increases genomic stability that prevents cancer
- Eliminates waste from the body
- Increases neuroendocrine homeostasis
- Decreases inflammation
- Increases lifespan
- Eliminates aging cells
- Improves muscle performance

Does Autophagy Help Women? how?

The ghrelin or the hunger hormone increases more quickly in women than in men. Women start feeling hungry again quickly after having a meal. Their bodies start craving food much faster and, therefore, are under more stress to look for energy sources. The cleansing of their body cells makes them less immune to catching diseases and helps them to develop a stronger immune system.

Does Autophagy Have Anti-Aging Effects Too?

Consider a real-life example. Assume that you have two cars, X and Y. You are somehow biased towards car X, and so you take much better care of it. You wash it every day, get it serviced every few months, and refuel the tank. But car Y does not see many bright days. It is just a backup option for you for the days X is out for servicing or repairs. You do not get its tank refueled, it stays covered in dirt and has been for just one servicing in years.

Now, which car do you think would last longer? Obviously, car X. When you pay attention to health and get the repairs done on time, faults and damages do not pile up. Your car X would stay as good as new even after years of driving, but car Y would start causing trouble very soon.

The same thing happens with the cells in your body. When the non-functional components and cellular waste keeps sitting inside the cell, it degrades your health and makes you look older. But when they keep recycling and renewing, it shows on your skin. Rejuvenated and youthful cells make your skin softer and healthier.

Autophagy is like a cellular garbage disposal system. Newer cells wash away the dead and unhealthy ones. This leads to increased elimination of aging cells. Autophagy slows down the aging mechanism of your body that makes you look younger and healthier for a long time.

How Does Your Body Renew Itself Through Autophagy?

Small things matter, and when it comes to aging, small things are the only ones that matter. Cells are what keep you healthy and sick. They store energy, carry oxygen and do everything for your body. And they are the ones that keep you from aging on the inside and outside.

Let us understand how this works. The cells in your body are continuously at work, so they experience a lot of wear and tear. The over-used cells eventually stop working, thus becoming useless. When this happens, the production of new and healthy cells is also discouraged by the useless ones.

These used up cells are known as senescent cells. A senescent cell is a living cell, but its functioning does not contribute to maintaining person's health. And while they do not contribute to anything, they do not let new cells to get formed in the body either. Over the years, the senescent cells keep accumulating in the body. They perform just baseline functions, stop the creation of new cells and promote inflammation. The worst part for women is that they speed up the aging of the nearby cells.

Autophagy clears away the damaged cells, thus making way for the youthful cells to appear. You stay young, healthy and energetic for a long period. Therefore, working towards burning up the waste in your body cells is a great thing for you to do.

Developing healthy habits in your life is a good way to live. No one likes an untidy home; while a shining home with new furniture is loved by all, including the ones who live there. Autophagy is a way to throw away all the old things from home and make space for refreshing new things.

Chapter 11.
The differences between fasting for men and for women

Men and women are different. There are subtle differences that are not only physical but emotional and mental between the two genders. Therefore, measuring them both with the same yardstick can become problematic.

The biggest thing that makes the treatment of women differently than men imperative is their ability to bear offspring's. This requires a special body and hormonal structuring and makes all the difference. Therefore, you can talk about all the equality, feminism and all those things, but nothing should undermine the fact that women have a different physical and hormonal structure that needs special attention.

Women have been entrusted with the responsibility to bear kids. The whole process of bearing kids, making it, and providing the required nutrition is heavily fat dependent. A woman's body gets prepared to bear a child as soon as it hits puberty. The body doesn't understand the legal restraints, and it always tries to remain in a state of readiness to bear kids. Till you hit menopause, either you want to have kids or not, your body would always try to attract fat so that whenever conception takes place, it is able to bear a healthy child. This need for readiness makes a substantial difference in the feeding needs of men and women.

Physiologically speaking a woman's body has higher body fat percentage than men. While a man may have an ideal essential body fat ratio of 3-5%, the women may have it anywhere between 10-13%. Even in athletes, male body fat ratio lies between 6-13% whereas female body fat ratio can be as high as 14-20%. In average body type men, the body fat ratio should fall between 18-24%. This ratio in women is between 25-31%. The reason for showing these stats is simple. It is important for women to understand that having a little higher body fat ratio is not only normal but natural. This is how their bodies have been designed. All those women, who are obsessed with zero figures or other such dimensions may be putting their natural body cycle at risk. Therefore, whenever a woman thinks of losing weight, this fact should be kept in mind.

Another thing that mandates that women have a different fasting schedule than men is their hormonal system. The hormonal cycle of women is highly sensitive to hunger signals. They are more sensitive to starvation, and their bodies are designed to bear kids, and that cannot be possible when there is a shortage of food. Therefore, longer and difficult fasts would hurt your fertility and childbearing abilities.

- This makes it necessary that women always move ahead with fasting schedules very slowly.
- They should never start with longer food gaps without practice.
- They must always increase their fasting period in small progression.
- They should not be adamant about continuing fasting for the complete duration. If there is a strong craving, they should end their fast that day and begin fresh the next day again.

· Women shouldn't keep fasts longer than 24 hours as that can seriously mess up their hormonal cycle.

If these things are followed, even women can follow intermittent fasting easily.

Effect of Fasting on the Hormonal System of Women

Fasting tells the body it isn't a good time for fertility. When you fast for long, and your body starts having an energy deficit on a consistent level, it starts conserving the energy for necessary functions and fertility is not one among them. This has been proven through several studies that prolonged fasting can lead to shrinking of ovaries.

However, it is important to clarify here that these experiments have only been conducted on mice. The induced fasting time was only of a few days, but on the life scale of mice, it could have meant fasting for much longer.

However, besides everything else, it is an undisputed fact that fasting for long is a problem for women. There are several hormones that get affected. The estrogen levels get messed up if the fasting is not done carefully or calorie restriction is carried out.

Here, it is again important to clarify that this imbalance can happen with any calorie restriction followed by women. It means regardless of the method followed like diet, calorie restriction or intermittent fasting, such problems can arise if due attention is not paid to the process.

Imbalance in the hormonal levels can have a wide impact. The practitioners may face metabolic disorders, weight loss ability, mood, bone density, energy, cognitive function, anxiety, and stress levels all may get affected.

Impact of starvation on various hormonal balances would be:

Impact of estrogen imbalance

- ✓ Low energy
- ✓ Poor heart health
- ✓ Infertility
- ✓ Poor glucose regulation
- ✓ Weight gain
- ✓ Reduced skin and hair health
- ✓ Poor cognitive function
- ✓ Decreased bone density
- ✓ Poor muscle tone

Imbalance can also trip the Cortisol levels in your body. It is the stress hormone. The impact would be:

- ✓ Sugar cravings
- ✓ Low energy
- ✓ Anxiety
- ✓ Fatigue
- ✓ Insomnia

Thyroid imbalance can also take place. It may lead to:

- ✓ Weight gain
- ✓ Brain fog
- ✓ Depression
- ✓ Anxiety
- ✓ Dry hair dry skin
- ✓ Irregular periods
- ✓ The feeling of cold or hot flashes

Fasting is a very healthy practice. Intermittent fasting is an even improvised version of fasting to eliminate the harmful things so that only beneficial things can be retained. However, incorrect observation of any procedure will lead to negative fallouts. Therefore, it is important that women should follow intermittent fasting in the right way and very carefully. They need to be more observant about the changes and never become lax in their approach.

Fasting tells the body it isn't a good time for fertility. When you fast for long, and your body starts having an energy deficit on a consistent level, it starts conserving the energy for necessary functions and fertility is not one among them. This has been proven through several studies that prolonged fasting can lead to shrinking of ovaries. Although the same impact has been visible even in male subjects. However, it is important to clarify here that these experiments have only been conducted on mice. The induced fasting time was only of a few days, but on the life scale of mice, it could have meant fasting for much longer.

Essential Things for Women to Keep in Mind While Practicing Intermittent Fasting

The most important thing for women to do to become successful in their intermittent fasting pursuit is to avoid giving 'starvation signals'. It sends the body into panic mode all of a sudden. The production of hunger hormones shoots up, and the body fiercely starts protecting the fat. In such cases, losing fat would become very challenging.

You can avoid all this very easily by following the things given below:

Don't Test the Limits

You must never try to stretch the fasting too far. You have to fast and then give your body the time to recover. If you are beginning fasting, never fast on consecutive days. Always allow your body the time to recover.

Don't Fast Too Long

Initially, you should begin by creating safe gaps between your meals. Eliminate snacks completely. Then try to stretch the gap between the meals a bit. When you fast at night, always ensure that the highest amount of time spent without food is at the beginning of the fast. It means it is always better to begin fasts early in the evening as you will not feel hungry. Stretching your fast for too long in the morning wouldn't be a very bright idea. In any case, the fasting duration should be anywhere between 12-14 hours only. Several studies have shown that women get much better results with comparatively shorter fasts than men.

No HIIT on Fasting Days

High-intensity interval training is an energy-demanding activity. It should be avoided at all costs on the fasting days, especially if you are beginning your intermittent fasting. It can drain you and create strong energy demands.

No Fasting During the Menstrual Cycle

There is significant blood loss during the periods, and your body needs a lot of rest. Your hormones are also going crazy during this time. Therefore, you must not practice intermittent fasting at this time.

Have a Healthy Diet

Food choices are very important in the case of women as their nutritional requirements are high. You must choose a very healthy diet full of all the nutrients so that your hormones remain in check.

When To Stop

- You should stop fasting if you notice the following things:
- Irregular periods or complete absence of periods
- Sudden resurfacing of sleep disorders without any apparent reason
- On facing sudden and drastic metabolic and digestive issues
- On experiencing sudden mood swings and brain fog
- On having sudden changes in the color of the skin or hair texture

Intermittent Fasting is NOT for You If:

- You have eating disorders
- Have got pregnant or trying to conceive

· Have sleep disorders

· Have adrenal fatigue

· You are suffering from PMS, PCOS, PCOD, Fibroids, Endometriosis, or other hormonal issues

How to Manage Hunger

Hunger pangs in women have great significance. They begin as a damage control mechanism. They can force you to break any resolve. The trick always is to ditch that hunger response and not to dodge it. There is a big difference between both.

You'll be fine as long as you are not feeling hungry, suppressing hunger to a great extent wouldn't be beneficial. You can do this by following some simple things:

Eat Nutrient Dense Food

It is very, very important that women eat a nutrient-dense diet while they are practicing intermittent fasting. A nutrient-dense diet doesn't let a vacuum of nutrients get created inside you as that can toss your hormones out of control. You will already be facing a shortfall of energy at times in a day. Do not also try to create a shortage of calories and nutrients.

It is very imperative to understand that if you are following intermittent fasting, you will lose fat and weight. You don't need to reduce your calorie or nutrient intake for that. Following any calorie-restrictive diet while following intermittent fasting will only harm your health. You must never do that. Here, two negatives wouldn't make a positive; it doesn't work like that.

Always go for a nutrient-dense diet. Forget the number of calories you would be consuming as nothing would go for storage and either it would be used or expelled. Moving only with this understanding can help you. Eat your fill up to your heart's content. The only condition should be to eat healthy and nutritious things and avoid junk foods.

Emphasize on Fats

Here, it will suffice to say that a fat-rich diet will help you in keeping the hunger signals suppressed. It will make your fasting easier.

Avoid Intense Workouts on Fasting Days

You should avoid intense exercise on the fasting days. Exercise on the non-fasting days and allow your body to recover on the fasting days.

Don't Remain Fixated on Fat Loss

Your main aim should always be good health and remember that if your body is healthy, there would always be a fat loss as your body wouldn't want to carry fat that is not bringing anything good. All the fat on our body gets accumulated as the body is facing extreme stress and chronic inflammation. Once these problems are resolved, the fat would go away on your own. You focus should always be to get healthy, and you'd get in shape automatically.

Keep Yourself Busy

On fasting days, it is important to remain busy. If you are sitting idle, then most of the time, only food will be playing at the back of your head. Read, write, enjoy with friends or family, or do some work. The aim should be to remain occupied as then the mind would go the least towards the thought of food.

Take Hunger Suppressors

You can take unsweetened black tea, coffee, fresh lime water with a pinch of salt if you feel the hunger pangs. These things can also help you in keeping hunger at bay. However, there is no need to fight with the hunger pangs a lot as you can start fresh again the next day.

Chapter 12.
Fasting for people over 50

Pros and cons for over 50

Side effects of intermittent fasting can be fatigue or headache. If you find these symptoms in yourself, it is best to clarify with a doctor whether and how you should practice one of the fasting methods.

It is also important for intermittent fasting that you eat a healthy and balanced diet during the phases in which you can eat. If you consume fewer calories than usual through Lent, it is all the more important that they come from nutrient-rich foods and provide you with all the nutrients you need.

Weight loss takes longer with intermittent fasting than with therapeutic fasting, but - as explained above - is sustainable and healthy. Of course, there is no weight loss if large amounts of unhealthy food are consumed on the eating days or during the eating times, one does not move, etc.

Pros

- Reduction of body fat (KFA)
- Improvement of cellular regeneration (keyword: anti-aging)
- Increased release of growth hormones
- Improved immune defense
- Lowering blood pressure
- Reduction of oxidative stress

- Prevention against diseases of civilization widespread in our society (diabetes, Cancer, high blood sugar, etc.)
- 30% increase in life expectancy (animal studies)

All in all, it can be said that eating food for a limited time is good for both health and appearance. But let's talk - we can do it among us - Tacheles: improved immune defense, reduced blood pressure and reduced oxidative stress in all honor, but what really drives us to do without one or more of our beloved meals every day is the prospect of a defined, athletic and above all aesthetic body

Cons

As with everything in life, there are of course two sides to the same coin when it comes to intermittent fasting. The change in eating rhythm, especially in the early days, can lead to increased feelings of hunger , reduced performance, nervousness, mood swings and, in extreme cases (e.g. in midsummer), also to weakness attacks.

In addition, there is a risk that IF supporters literally and regularly "overeat" during the permitted eight hours of food intake. Of course it is completely legitimate to celebrate the successfully completed fasting phase with a feast - after all, people have been looking for it long enough. However - and this is now a crucial point - excessive gluttony will very likely only lead to an increase in calories at the end of the day. And a plus in the calorie balance automatically leads to a weight gain - unfortunately we all know it all too well.

The good news: If you carefully introduce your body to the new eating habits and don't regularly take it to the (calorie) top, ninety-nine percent and nine percent of the "contras" just mentioned are already obsolete anyway

Advantages of intermittent fasting for over 50

The advantages of intermittent fasting at a glance:

* Promotes fat loss
* Is considered an anti-aging agent
* No feeling of abandonment, strict diet rules and prohibitions
* Learn again to pay attention to your own feeling of hunger
* Digestion is relieved
* No counting calories or demonizing a single macronutrient
* Suitable for office and everyday use
* No great planning or previous knowledge necessary
* Reduces cravings
* Many health benefits such as lower risk of cancer, diabetes, cardiovascular diseases, better blood values, longer life expectancy, less inflammation in the body
* Increased mental performance, clarity
* Permanent diet on request

Disadvantages of intermittent fasting for over 50

As always, the same applies to intermittent fasting: not everything that glitters is gold.

* Freeze due to low blood pressure
* Hunger, moodiness
* listlessness

* Indigestion such as flatulence, heartburn or constipation

* Dizziness

* Fatigue and increased yawning

* Restlessness

* Tremble

* Sweat

* Reduced performance during sports due to low blood pressure

* Risk of missing all the positive effects of the fasting period through uncontrolled or unhealthy eating due to the lack of rules for the eating phase

* Less spontaneity and flexibility in everyday life (for example when spontaneously inviting meals during the fasting phase or when you bring a cake with you to the office)

* Fasting too often (more than three days a week) can lead to protein deficiency , especially for athletes , or at least to insufficient protein intake to build new muscles (in the worst case, even muscle breakdown)

How intermittent fasting works

Depending on the concept, the different methods of intermittent fasting differ slightly, but the basics are the same for everyone: Fixed periods of time in which you can eat what and how much you want alternate with those in which you fast. Important: The fasting period must always be longer than the period in which eating is allowed. The twelve-hour fast is the minimum: Only then should the body's own glycogen stores in the liver and muscles be used up and the body switches to burning fat like "correct" therapeutic fasting. In this phase you also have to be really strict and really not allowed to eat or drink anything. Only water, black coffee and unsweetened and are allowed green tea. Even a small sip of milk in morning coffee is taboo, as this would raise blood sugar and stimulate insulin production.

All the better: Everything is allowed in the meal phase. Intermittent fasting is therefore not a diet with too many regulations on WHAT you can eat, but WHEN you can eat. Of course, it is still recommended that you follow the rules for a healthy diet, especially if you want to use intermittent fasting to lose weight.

You are also free to choose how many meals you eat in the allowed hours. However, not too many are recommended and especially the snack should be deleted. Ultimately, this decision remains with Intermittent fasting is up to you.

If you want to try interrupted fasting, there are three basic rules for you:

* Find out which of the intermittent options works best for you. Your choice depends on how long you can do well without food. The different forms differ in frequency and duration of the food restriction.
* Only water or unsweetened beverages such as coffee or tea are allowed during the fasting phase. During this time, the body gets everything it needs from your reserves.
* The rest of the time, you can eat as normal. Except for the usual recommendations for a healthy diet - i.e. little refined sugar, not eating too much and too late, preferably no fast food - there are no guidelines.

* Depending on the individual goals and preferences, different forms of intermittent fasting are possible, which differ in their ratio of fasting to mealtime.

Benefits of Intermittent Fasting for over 50

At the beginning of the fasting phase, the glycogen stores (storage of glucose) of the liver and muscles are mobilized. If these are empty, fat is broken down. The free fatty acids are then converted to ketones and used to generate energy.

Proteins are also used to provide energy, especially in the first days of fasting. Then the body increasingly uses depot fat. Abdominal fat (visceral fat tissue), which is harmful to health, is used primarily to generate energy. It is particularly metabolically active and sends out hormones and inflammation factors, which then promote cardiovascular diseases or the development of cancer. Part of the desired effects of fasting result from the reduction in abdominal fat.

Due to the increased energy production and metabolism of ketones, the organism is burdened with acid. Sufficient drinking and physical activity are crucial so that acid excretion can be boosted by the kidneys and the acetone formed can be exhaled. The fruity bad breath is characteristic of the burning of ketone bodies.

A ketogenic diet (low carbohydrate intake, hence the metabolism of fats to ketone bodies) protects nerve cells from certain damaging influences. This has a protective effect on various nerve diseases, such as Parkinson's disease or dementia. The ketone bodies could have the same effect when fasting.

Long-term fasting has a positive effect on rheumatoid arthritis. Through preventive fasting numerous risk factors for aging and age-related diseases are reduced. Weight, systolic blood pressure, total body and abdominal fat decreased. In addition, fasting blood sugar, C-reactive protein (inflammation marker) and LDL cholesterol improved. This suggests a preventive effect on the development of various clinical pictures, such as diabetes mellitus type II or cardiovascular diseases. Preventive fasting has so far hardly been researched.

Chapter 13.
Tips to Get Started

Whether this is your first fast or your thousandth, everyone sometimes needs a little boost to get started.

1. Choose a method that aligns with your daily routine! Go easy on yourself! Choose what feels like a natural extension of your daily routine. Your body, mind, and soul will thank you for it!

2. Plan your method! Don't go into your first Intermittent Fast (or yours fifth, for that matter!) without planning which method you'll choose, based on your lifestyle, routines, and tendencies.

3. Stick with your chosen method at least for the first week! You might feel tired of what you've chosen, and you might feel equally frustrated that things aren't working for you right away. But if you dedicate at least a week with a method, you can be sure whether or not it's helpful (and if not, you can discern how to tweak it to be better).

4. Do the research! If there's something else you've heard of (a rumor, a method, a fact, etc.) that are not included in this book, go find it! Research any questions that arise to be sure what you choose is right for you.

5. If you're unsure, check with your doctor or nutritionist! There are a lot of complexities involved with Intermittent Fasting, and one of the biggest complexities is the conundrum of your body. Your doctor or nutritionist will know your body and its

needs best, so if you've decided on a method, run it by them to be sure that it's the one for you.

6. Alter your diet slightly ahead of time! If you're going to do a day-on, day-off style of fasting, start by cutting out snacks! Scale back what you're eating to make things easier on yourself when you start. On the other hand, if you're pairing diet with IF, start the diet before you start fasting so that you have a handle on that better (and so that you don't have to detox from certain foods while you're also fasting).

7. Check the nutrients you'll be receiving! Before you fast, make sure you're looking at the macronutrient levels of the foods you'll be eating. You want to make sure you have the right number of calories, carbs, proteins, and fats to stay healthy and energized.

8. Before the first day, make sure you're prepared! On the evening before your fast, make your dinner choice as conscious as possible, down to the timing. Don't gorge yourself and don't go crazy on something overly rich or decadent. Instead, eat a modest dinner that's not too late and not too filling. Furthermore, don't snack after dinner so that you can wake up with a decent chunk of your fast already underway.

9. Keep a lot of drinks on hand! Drinks will be pivotal for keeping your energy and spirits up, so make sure you have them and that they're the right types of drinks to support IF!.

10. To establish a routine, take things slow and don't be too hard on yourself! It can be hard to adjust to a whole new food-related lifestyle, so don't push yourself too hard too soon into

the process. Stay realistic with your expectations for yourself and the fast.

What to Expect

When you start Intermittent Fasting, you'll want to keep several things in mind so that you know exactly what to expect.

First, you'll want to expect mornings to be a whole new adventure. Sometimes, (based on the method you choose) your mornings will be slow and stagnant, and sometimes they'll be filled with energy. Sometimes, you may be super hungry in the morning, while other times you might be perfectly fine.

Second, expect that coffee will become your new best friend. Coffee will help you snap some energy when you're feeling low without food, and it can also keep you focused on something to do with your hands and mouth when you feel hungry but can't quite eat yet due to timing.

Third, expect that your first week might be rough and moody. You might have to build up a tolerance to all that Intermittent Fasting has to offer, but once you cross that first hurdle, you should have a much easier time moving on.

Fourth, some things in your life will increase. You'll become more present, more mindful, more conscious of the world and your feelings, and more conscious of how food makes you feel as well as what it makes you do and say.

Fifth, some things in your life will decrease, namely your weight! You could also see a decrease in sleep for the first few weeks, and while you go through the body's initial detoxification period, you might also find that your sleep isn't restful even when you can get it. Eventually, things will even out, and sleep will not be an issue anymore.

Sixth, you will get cranky and emotional in the first few weeks. During this period, you will be going through heavy detoxification of body and mind. You'll have to push through any anxiety, temper tantrums, and restlessness to keep your mind on the prize. You may even get a little smelly during this time as you sweat out all the bad, but your body and mind will thank you for this later!

Seventh, and finally, expect that your relationship with food will completely change for the better. You will be less of a slave to your cravings and desires, and you will be more understanding of people who live with less. You will be less dependent, more informed, more grateful, and less hangry when food takes a while.

While some of these expectations are relatively negative, most if not all have incredibly positive potential. Once you're through the first few weeks of your fast, you should see the silver lining of each expectation clearly.

What to Look Out For

All the above expectations should end up relatively resolved after the first week, but there will be signs in your body if things are not resolved and getting worse. These signs will be things to look out for, and if the situations don't improve with alteration and time, it may mean that IF isn't right for you after all. However, keep these tidbits in mind for your practice so that you can be on the lookout for your own best interest.

First, watch out if you experience constant headaches, lightheadedness, or dizziness. If you have these experiences just once or twice, that can be resolved, but if these arise constantly, there's a deeper problem that needs to be addressed.

Second, and furthermore, if you're overly tired without the ability to sleep or constantly sleeping after the second week, there's something wrong with your method or the way you're going about it.

Third, watch out if you're getting hunger pangs that can't be dealt with. Generally, during Intermittent Fasting, you'll experience hunger, and that's normal. You'll ride through the hunger wave and move past it. However, if these waves come again and again with no satiation, you might be in a bit of trouble.

Fourth, and finally, watch for any severe personality changes. If you start becoming obsessively compelled to practice your fast in new ways or if you feel that you're becoming overly controlling of or controlled by your fast, it might be time to take a break.

As always, it's your body, so it's your choice. Just make sure it's the smartest and most informed choice you're capable of making.

Chapter 14.
Exercising During an Intermittent Fast

One of the most interesting aspects of the scientific research into intermittent fasting comes in the theory that intermittent fasting is actually the best way to maintain muscle mass while you lose weight. We tend to think of muscles as beasts that need to be constantly fed in order to maintain their stature – but in reality, all muscles are scar tissue! Your giant biceps are the result of microscopic muscle tears healing over and over again, forming scar tissue, and growing as a result. Your muscles do need a decent amount of protein and calcium, but most of these fuel sources are for the biological processes your body enacts on your muscles. And anyway, scientific studies demonstrate again and again that eating regularly after a period of fasting promotes weight loss, but not the same amount of muscle loss. When you chose to take on an intermittent fast, you might become worried about losing the muscle you've already built. This happens with most diets, especially if you don't pay close attention to making sure you're eating and working out for muscle growth. You already know that intermittent fasting helps your body produce that miracle chemical, human growth hormone, in much higher doses. Human growth hormone helps to promote the growth of strong, lean muscle, while also shutting down that part of your biological starvation mechanism that tells you to use your own body for fuel. However. There are a few things to take into consideration when you're working out on an intermittent fast. First of all, you simply don't have the same caloric input to fuel your regular energy output. There's just no way that you will be able to do that same exact workout on a fasting day that you would on a non-fasting day without sending at least a few of your muscles into fatigue. In order to balance the days when you're fasting with a gym workout, you should try and focus on strength training, flexibility training, and gentle low-intensity cardio. While these all surely aren't the high-intensity lifting sessions you might be used to, they're still important exercises to keeping your body fit. Since you can't produce the same catabolic output as you would on an eating day, you have to make sure that you're working within the confines of what your body can do (if you're eating on an intermittent fast that doesn't have you fast for more than sixteen hours, remember, this doesn't really count.) When you fast, you should stick to exercises like yoga and Pilates that can engage your muscles on a much smaller scale than would a bench press or Russian deadlift.

Instead, you get to focus more on control and endurance – which are two essential parts of being a well-rounded athlete. You're perfectly welcome to take time on an intermittent fast for long, sustained intensity cardio as well if you don't tend to lean towards flexibility.

Chapter 15.
Myths About Intermittent Fasting

There are many myths out there about Intermittent Fasting. the common myths are as follows;

MYTH: Your body will definitely enter in starvation mode.

TRUTH: Your body will not definitely enter in starvation mode through Intermittent Fasting. Skipping meals or adjusting to longer periods between meals where you don't eat is not going to make you starve. It's going to help your body remember how to absorb nutrients. It's going to help you thrive instead.

MYTH: You'll lose muscle in this endeavor.

TRUTH: This myth goes along the same lines as the first one, above. Just like your body won't enter the starvation mode (unless something goes very, very wrong or you're trying to do too much); your body won't lose muscle through IF. The only reason why intermittent fasting would cause muscle loss would be if it was causing you to starve, but once again, the first myth addresses this falsity, making this myth false as well.

MYTH: You'll almost assuredly overeat during eating windows, and that's not healthy at all.

TRUTH: While some people will have the instinct to overeat during eating windows, not everyone will overeat. Even those who do at the start will realize how to move forward without this overeating instinct in the future. Your body will urge you to overeat because, at the start, it won't realize what you're doing to it, but as long as you keep portion sizes largely the same and don't gorge on snacks, your body will adjust and so will your appetite.

MYTH: Your metabolism will slow down dangerously.

TRUTH: Your metabolism won't slow down just because you're eating less often. People who think this myth is true, only assume that restricted caloric intake will make one's metabolism slow down over time, but these individuals forget that IF isn't necessarily about cutting down calories overall. It's actually about cutting down the times during which one consumes calories. There needn't be any caloric restriction whatsoever! It just depends on the practitioner and what he or she decides to do with dieting in addition to IF.

MYTH: You'll only gain weight if you try skipping meals.

TRUTH: This myth is based on the same logic that drives the myth about overeating. If you gorge yourself during your eating windows, you'll surely gain weight, but hardly anyone will continuously gorge with IF. Anyone who tries will realize how unsuccessful it is, so he or she will not continuously gorge in response. Anyone who doesn't realize his or her efforts with eating are unsuccessful will soon realize that something's wrong, as his or her weight shows no improvement. Skipping meals never necessarily means that someone will gain weight. It just means that people who skip meals and gorge or overeat when it is mealtime won't see the desired effects.

MYTH: During fast periods, you literally can't eat anything.

TRUTH:This myth is partially true and partially false. It's true only for methods like 12:12, 14:10, 16:8, and 20:4 that require fasting and eating in alternation within each individual day. For 12:12 method, for example, you'd spend 12 hours fasting and 12 hours eating. In this case, you would definitely not eat anything or consume any calories during that 12-hour fasting window, but the same isn't true for methods that alternate between days "on" and days "off" between fasting and eating. For those types of methods, you absolutely can eat during fasting periods! It might feel counterintuitive as you read these words, but you don't explicitly have to eat nothing during fast periods. Most methods that have full days of fasting actually allow for caloric intake as long as it's restricted by 20-25% of one's normal intake. Therefore, for methods like 5:2, alternate-day, eat-stop-eat, and crescendo, on days when you're fasting, you can still consume around 500 calories, and that will help a lot!

MYTH: There's only one way to do IF that's right and truly the best.

TRUTH: This myth is absolutely and utterly false. There is no one right way to practice Intermittent Fasting, and part of the beauty of IF is that there are so many different methods, meaning each approaching IF likely has a few different options to choose from. Similarly, different body and personality types will be drawn to different methods, based on individuals' abilities and goals. IF is about flexibility, adjustment, and self-correction. There's no one right method for everyone, and there's no "best" method to strive for. Do whatever method feels right and suits your life, and once you've found it, practice it as long as you can! That's far more realistic and accessible.

MYTH: It's not natural to fast like that.

TRUTH: It's more natural to practice Intermittent Fasting than it is to eat three full meals each day! It's more connected to our evolutionary drives and to our primitive selves to eat like this. And it's better for our brains, hearts, cells, and digestive systems to have a break from food once in a while to recalibrate. As you learned in the Introduction, people have been practicing Intermittent Fasting as long as humans have been in existence. It's only myths like this that circulate today that make it seem like IF is foreign, unhealthy, and dangerous. Animals of all types become healthier after periods of fasting, and humans are no different. Remember that we are animals and that IF is in our nature. Proceed with that confidence and knowledge!

Q & A

To wrap things up, this section is all about those final questions that might linger in your mind. It's about addressing your concerns and putting your mind at ease. If you have a question that doesn't appear to be answered anywhere in this book, ask to your trusted nutritionist and make sure to do things right.

15 Questions & Answers about IF

Whether they're about methods, strategies, approaches, measurements of success, or otherwise, these questions (and their respective answers) should address any lingering concerns or confusions for any future (or current) IF practitioners.

1. Who is Intermittent Fasting for?

IF is actually for anyone! It works best for people who are simply serious about making their health better and about changing their weights for the better without sacrificing their diets.

2. What should I consider before my first fast?

Think of your bodily limitations, your daily routine, your work schedule, and your tendencies with hunger and thirst. The more you know about yourself, the better! On the other hand, the more you know about the method you're going to try, the better, too! Consider every detail you can, from your personality to your body weight, your tendencies, your cravings, and more. Together, all these details will help you make your first fast the best and most lasting change in your life.

3. If I'm diabetic, should I try IF?

Absolutely! Give IF a try, but don't be too strict with diet or exercise while you attempt it. Additionally, don't be too strict with your timing or snack restriction. Diabetic individuals can experience troubles with IF when they limit themselves too much, so make sure you're not sacrificing your health but definitely give it a try!

4. Will IF help with more than weight loss?

Yes, definitely! Intermittent Fasting can heal the brain, the heart, the digestive system, the mood, and so much more! It's not just about weight loss, and anyone who insists it is just lying to you.

5. Which method of IF is best?

The answer to this question is more subjective than objective. There's no one method that's best for everyone. In fact, each individual should choose the method that works best for him or her based on the guidelines listed in chapter 6.

6. Where should I begin if I'm interested in IF?

Start by doing some reading! Research IF and see what it can do for you. Then, start making the simple steps to your own IF transition. These simple steps include snacking less, eating less often late at night, waiting a little longer to eat in the morning, and making sure to eat dinner a little bit earlier.

7.   I'm breastfeeding—should I try IF or wait until I'm done?

Great question! Generally, I suggest you waiting until you're done breastfeeding to try IF or to reinstate it again. While you're breastfeeding, your body needs a specific subset of nutrients to produce what your baby needs. With an intense exercise regimen and practice of caloric restriction, you may do more harm to your body and your baby than good. It's not worth the risk, but as I wrote above, there's a possibility.

8.   Should I exercise while I try IF?

As you transition into IF, start by trying to exercise occasionally, but don't expect that you'll be able to exercise as much as you had been without IF. Start small and build up to see what your body can handle, given the restricted intake. Women and diabetic individuals are almost exclusively recommended to not exercise while attempting IF. The consequences are too problematic for me to want you to push those boundaries.

9.   Should I diet while I try IF?

You can certainly try! However, most people will realize that strict dieting does not pair all that well with IF unless it's the Keto Diet. People who diet by calorie counting will not benefit by taking this strategy into IF. People who diet by restricting protein or fat will equally not benefit with IF. Therefore, if you do combine dieting and IF, make sure your diet isn't too strict, and leave wiggle room for growth and troubleshooting. If you're attempting the Keto Diet, with its helpful divisions of fat, protein, and carbs, you may find that your diet is perfect for IF. As always, take things one day at a time, and don't cling too harshly to your diet! There may be times when it helps, but there will be times when it doesn't. Just stay open to changes and fluctuations in your experience.

10. I'm working on IF right now—why do I have a headache constantly?

Not everyone feels this type of head pain while fasting, but it is more often women than men that go through this experience. Due to studies done on Islamic peoples observing Ramadan, we can tell that the cause to this pain is not always dehydration. In fact, it's much more related to the kind of headache one gets after quitting coffee drinking. Essentially, it's a withdrawal symptom from something, and it will fade and go away after you keep practicing the fast. If it doesn't go away, it might be time to stop (see chapter 9).

11. Is it okay to drink during IF or is it strictly no intake?

It's absolutely acceptable (and even recommended!) for individuals to drink during fast periods. Just try to make sure your drink has no calories (so no soda, not a lot of juice, etc.), and you should be aligned with your goals! Simply remember that fasting periods are supposed to be times of rest for your body and mind, so you won't want to add anything too intense to that bodily mix in these moments. Keep the calories of the drink low, and you'll be set.

12. If I take supplements and vitamins each day, should I stop them while trying IF?

The short answer to this question is yes. The longer answer to this question is that you might want to hold off on taking your supplements on days when you're fully fasting. However, if you're not doing day-on, day-off fasts but fasting and eating within each day instead, you should have no problem continuing to take all supplements daily, as you normally would.

13. Will IF screw up my metabolism?

Your metabolism is much more connected to your body fat than most people know and are taught. Therefore, all concerns over messing up one's metabolism through IF are largely unfounded. The truth is that as your body fat goes down, so will your metabolism. The less you have to burn, the less intensely your metabolism works, but that's all balanced out by the body's natural processes. Essentially, there's no way you can screw this up.

14. Is IF safe for pregnant women and expecting mothers?

Many different groups hotly debates this, but the gist of the answer is that it depends on the mother, the situation, and the advice of the mother's doctor. Sometimes, IF poses no threat, while other times it's disastrous. Err on the side of caution and speak with your doctor or nutritionist first.

15. I have hypothyroid. Should I try IF or not?

With hypothyroid, you should still be able to try IF! The trick for you will be to make sure you never fast for more than a day at a time. Your bodily rhythms will be greatly distressed if you attempt to fast more than 24 hours at once.

Conclusion

Although you won't be cutting out entire food groups while you're on an intermittent fast, it can still be incredibly beneficial to your energy levels to take a few supplements.

Even if you weren't about to begin a difficult fasting diet, the chances are high that you're deficient in more than a few of your essential vitamins and minerals. Vitamins and minerals, remember, are called your micronutrients, and they work hand in hand with your macronutrients (carbohydrates, proteins, and fats) to make sure you can use energy, build proteins, and execute life processes inside your body. If you aren't getting enough micronutrients in your diet during a non-fasting day, you might not feel as good as you could or lose as much weight as you could, if you had a decent supply of them.

The daily micronutrients that your body needs range from the beloved and familiar – vitamin D, vitamin C, calcium, and potassium – to more obscure and lesser-known minerals like zinc, thiamin, and magnesium. While your multivitamin might be able to give you certain boosts of each, you should pay attention to the nutritional contents of each multivitamin to make sure. Outside of a comprehensive vitamin, you should begin to supplement your intermittent fasting diet with five to seven of these essential micronutrients. If you didn't already know, calcium doesn't just facilitate the growth and maintenance of strong bones. Calcium is also essential for the movement of all of your muscles, every time you move. Calcium facilitates the contraction and relaxing of your muscles, which means that you should probably supplement it alongside your intermittent fasting schedule if you plan on working out. Making gains on an intermittent fasting diet already requires more focus than a normal workout routine, and oftentimes you'll get a potassium supplement alongside your calcium as a helping hand for absorption into your bloodstream. Alongside your calcium supply, you should also aim to increase your magnesium before going on an intermittent fast. Magnesium is a mineral that helps our overall brain function. This micronutrient isn't limited to just strong cognitive processes, however. Magnesium also boosts your immune health, nerve function, and blood pressure. In fact, magnesium is so important to our bodies that if we find ourselves in low supply, our metabolism will start to harvest the magnesium from our bones. The next micronutrient you'll want to beef up on is your iron supply. Iron is a unique micronutrient in that your body which can build up a hefty supply that lasts for a while – but if you're already low, or you're a female and are predisposed to be anemic, you should supplement with iron tablets. You only have to take them for about one month, and you should consult with your doctor to ensure you take the right dosage. When you intermittent fast, you might also want to take something called a "branched-chain amino acid". Branched-chain amino acids are often used by athletes to facilitate strong recovery after a hard work out. While your muscles might feel the benefits of your increased human growth hormone, it's worth it to augment your muscle protection to make sure you don't lose mass. Even without an increased amount of human growth hormone, your body on a fast might sustain muscle loss naturally.

The last supplement that you'll want to add to your intermittent fasting routine is called beta-hydroxybutyrate. Beta-hydroxybutyrate is one of the three parts of a ketone body, the fuel source that your body relies on during a keto diet when you metabolize healthy fats. These supplements are also called "exogenous ketones", and they essentially help boost your body back into a state of strong ketosis. If you aren't eating on a solid ketogenic diet, you can take exogenous ketones in your diet to increase the likelihood that your body will burn the stored glucose still on your person. If you are eating on a solid ketogenic diet while fasting, exogenous ketones can make up for a day when you ate too many carbohydrates and know you might have set back your weight loss. Each one of these essential micronutrients can help boost your weight loss, energy, and muscle retention on an intermittent fast – but they're also things we need daily, in a regular supply. Even when you aren't dieting or trying to lose weight, supplementing your diet can bring you endless benefits that you didn't know you were missing.